D0828145

Respiratory Home Care
The Essentials

Respiratory Home Care
The Essentials

Patrick J. Dunne, MEd, RRT
President/Corporate General Partner
Southwest Medical Emporium
Fullerton, California

Susan L. McInturff, RCP, RRT
Staff Therapist
Farrell's Home Health
Bremerton, Washington

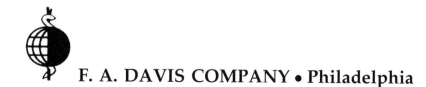

F. A. DAVIS COMPANY • Philadelphia

F. A. Davis Company
1915 Arch Street
Philadelphia, PA 19103

Copyright © 1998 by F. A. Davis Company

All rights reserved. This book is protected by copyright. No part of it may be reproduced, stored in a retrieval system, or transmitted in any form or by any means, electronic, mechanical, photocopying, recording, or otherwise, without written permission from the publisher.

Printed in the United States of America

Last digit indicates print number: 10 9 8 7 6 5 4 3

Publisher, Health Professions: Jean-François Vilain
Senior Editor: Lynn Borders Caldwell
Developmental Editor: Crystal Spraggins
Senior Production Editor: Roberta Massey
Cover Designer: Louis J. Forgione

As new scientific information becomes available through basic and clinical research, recommended treatments and drug therapies undergo changes. The authors and publisher have done everything possible to make this book accurate, up to date, and in accord with accepted standards at the time of publication. The authors, editors, and publisher are not responsible for errors or omissions or for consequences from application of the book, and make no warranty, expressed or implied, in regard to the contents of the book. Any practice described in this book should be applied by the reader in accordance with professional standards of care used in regard to the unique circumstances that may apply in each situation. The reader is advised always to check product information (package inserts) for changes and new information regarding dose and contraindications before administering any drug. Caution is especially urged when using new or infrequently ordered drugs.

Library of Congress Cataloging-in-Publication Data
Dunne, Patrick J., 1944–
    Respiratory home care: The essentials / Patrick J. Dunne, Susan
  L. McInturff.
        p.   cm.
    Includes bibliographical references and index.
    ISBN 0-8036-0154-9 (alk. paper)
        1. Respiratory organs—Diseases—Patients—Home care.
    2. Respiratory therapy.   I. McInturff, Susan L., 1955–
    II. Title.
        [DNLM: 1. Respiratory Therapy.   2. Home Care Services.   WF 145
    D923r   1998]
    RC735.H65D86   1998
    362.1'962—dc21
    DNLM/DLC
    for Library of Congress   97-18412
                                                                                              CIP

Authorization to photocopy items for internal or personal use, or the internal or personal use of specific clients, is granted by F. A. Davis Company for users registered with the Copyright Clearance Center (CCC) Transactional Reporting Service, provided that the fee of $.10 per copy is paid directly to CCC, 222 Rosewood Drive, Danvers, MA 01923. For those organizations that have been granted a photocopy license by CCC, a separate system of payment has been arranged. The fee code for users of the Transactional Reporting Service is: 8036-0154/98 0 + $.10.

Special thanks to the talented and dedicated staff at Southwest Medical, especially Jeff Franck, whose contributions and support made this undertaking possible. To my wife, Diane, and children, Jonathan and Christopher, your influence and motivation on my life have been more than you will ever know. Finally, without the early guidance and continued encouragement from my mother, Liz, this author's career in respiratory therapy would have ended long ago. Thanks again, Mom!

PJD

To Gerilynn and Dr. Hodgkin for getting me started; to Michael Iott for his help and perspective; and especially to my husband for his unwavering patience, support, and love.

SLM

Foreword

Historically, much of chronic care, particularly in patients with respiratory disease states, took place in the home. One needs only to tour Colorado Springs, Colorado, once a mecca for those suffering from chronic, unrelenting tuberculosis, to see the sun porches on many homes where patients spent most of their days trying to "catch the cure"—that combination of high altitude, sunshine, and nutritious diet that all later proved to be beneficial in arresting active tuberculosis. With the development of high-technology medicine, which requires organized hospital and intensive care units, care of patients with a variety of respiratory illnesses shifted to the hospitals. Although great strides have been made in the treatment of individuals who suffer from insults resulting in acute respiratory failure, many chronic patients remain who require home care service. Hospitals have greatly reduced the length of stay of all patients, mandating excellent home care services for respiratory patients. Without home care follow-up, readmission to the hospital is often indicated.

Our own experience in home care began in 1965 with our introduction to the first portable liquid oxygen system. After patients were proved to be physiologically and globally improved, they naturally went home with their oxygen supply. Working with the Visiting Nurse Association of Denver, we provided the initial home visits. Soon many people required home oxygen; some patients had the residuals of poliomyelitis and were on ventilators at home, but they did not have an organized system other than that provided by visiting nurses.

Today, the respiratory care practitioner (RCP) plays a key role in the home care of pulmonary patients. The home care RCP is trained in the pathophysiology of disease and the technology that helps mitigate these states, and he or she can understand firsthand why human suffering, anxiety, and despair plague the life and happiness of many who continue to struggle to breathe. Many patients can live happy, healthy, and productive lives with home-based respiratory care.

Respiratory home care is provided to patients of all ages and includes monitoring of patients on medical devices, psychosocial support, education, physical assessment, and a reporting system back to the referring physician.

Continuing education is necessary for patients with chronic conditions. Studies show that patients and caregivers forget most of the information taught during the emotional crisis of hospitalization. People learn better when they are not under stress. The patient's home is usually a place of comfort and security; therefore, home teaching is always necessary for the patient and family members.

Today, we should encourage the shift back to the home as the center of care for most chronic respiratory disorders. The RCP plays a key role in this evolution. Although perhaps not quite as exciting as intensive care medicine, home care can be more gratifying because it deals more intimately with the human aspects of care and often helps the patient return to health and a high quality of life. Home care is far more cost efficient than hospital care and, in the end, even more satisfying.

The RCP provides medical care, but equally important is the reassurance and continued education he or she provides the family members and the patient. The RCP usually is the first one to recognize a deterioration of health of the patient or the caregiver. Often this deterioration can be relieved by immediate attention before a crisis develops. In this regard the home care RCP plays an important role in preventive care.

We congratulate the authors, both of whom are highly experienced and qualified to have produced this magnificent volume. We hope that it will be a resource book for the next 100 years of home care and beyond.

Thomas L. Petty, MD
Professor of Medicine
Health Sciences Center
University of Colorado
Denver, Colorado

Louise M. Nett, RN, RRT
Information Specialist
HealthOne
Center for Health Sciences Education
Denver, Colorado

Preface

Respiratory care practitioners (RCPs) have been providing respiratory care services in the home setting for decades, but until recently "respiratory home care" has been viewed as a *site* of care rather than as a specialty area of practice. This all changed with the formation of the Home Care Specialty Section within the American Association for Respiratory Care in 1994. Prior to this momentous step, home care was largely looked on as a place for clinicians who were "burned out" from working in the more traditional acute care setting. The value of the home care RCP in the overall management of patients with chronic pulmonary disease went virtually unnoticed. Respiratory therapy educational programs were not graduating students whose career goals included home care; rather, students' goals following graduation were to go into either acute or neonatal critical care, management, or education. One might "retire" to home care if one did not leave the profession altogether.

How things have changed! Home care is now widely recognized as the fastest growing segment of the nation's health care delivery system. Further, with the notion of transitional care now firmly embedded as an integral part of health care restructuring, home care is viewed by many as the most appropriate manner to effectively manage most chronic medical conditions. For patients afflicted with chronic pulmonary diseases, their ability to receive optimum home care services is directly dependent on the availability of a competent, highly trained, and committed home care RCP. Time and experience have proved that there is no acceptable substitute. Indeed, then, the role (and value) of the home care RCP has never been greater, and the opportunities for professional and personal growth remain boundless.

This book is for respiratory therapy students and clinicians who are considering a career in health care *outside* the traditional acute care hospital. The main focus is obviously home respiratory care: the elements of a successful home visit, the various types of home respiratory equipment, pediatric home care, infection control, documentation, and reimbursement mechanics. A chapter on pulmonary rehabilitation is included because this is a specialty practice outside of the acute care setting in which a growing number of RCPs are finding employment. Moreover, many of the techniques used in pulmonary rehabilitation programs are likewise used by home care RCPs when evaluating and educating their pulmonary patients. A chapter on subacute respiratory care is likewise included because there is a growing link between subacute respiratory care and home respiratory care. In the future, as the role of the acute care hospital diminishes, many of the referrals received for home respiratory care are expected to emanate from subacute care settings.

As with most attempts to formalize a wide body of knowledge into a single compendium, one is always faced with the daunting challenge of what to leave in and what to leave out. As co-authors, our intention is to provide an overview of a rapidly growing segment of the health care delivery system that is largely misunderstood and underappreciated by the more mainstream practitioners. In that regard, we recognize that it would not be possible to provide an exhaustive treatment of every aspect and nuance of respiratory home care. Some readers, therefore, will find that the material is not as detailed as they would like. We hope that, in such situations, the reader pursues a more in-depth investigation of the citations provided at the end of each chapter. For others, we invite you to learn firsthand about the challenges, opportunities, and contributions that can accompany a successful regimen of home respiratory care and the skills and competencies required to become a member of this exciting and timely specialty.

Patrick J. Dunne, MEd, RRT
Susan J. McInturff, RCP, RRT

Contributors

Lia Shaw Miller, BA, RCP
Project Director
North Bay HICAP
Health Insurance Counseling and
  Advocacy Program
Petaluma, California

**Gerilynn L. Connors, RCP, RRT,
  BS, FAACVPR**
Director
Pulmonary Rehabilitation Clinical
  Coordinator
Nicotine Intervention Program
St. Helena Hospital
Deer Park, California

Patrick J. Dunne, MEd, RRT
President/Corporate General Partner
Southwest Medical Emporium
Fullerton, California

Michael McDonald, BS, RRT
Regional Vice President
Pediatric Services of America, Inc.
Denver, Colorado

Susan L. McInturff, RCP, RRT
Staff Therapist
Farrell's Home Health
Bremerton, Washington

**Charles McIntyre, CRTT, RCP,
  NPRCP**
Executive Director
National Network for Pediatric
  Homecare
Van Nuys, California

Janice Tucker, RCP, RRT
Area Manager
UPC Health Network
Spokane, Washington

Reviewers

Charles Carroll, EdD, RRT
Dean
Health Careers and Wellness
Daytona Beach Community College
Daytona Beach, Florida

Melanie A. Ciesielski, RRT
Educator
Respiratory Care Technology
Forsyth Technical Community
  College
Winston-Salem, North Carolina

Tammy P. Crump, MS, RRT
Program Director
Respiratory Care Program
Stanly Community College
Albemarle, North Carolina

Marie A. Fenske, EdD, RRT
Program Director
Respiratory Care Program
Gateway Community College
Phoenix, Arizona

Cynthia L. Howder, BS, RRT, CPFT
Program Director
Department of Respiratory Therapy
Seattle Central Community College
Seattle, Washington

Peter W. Kennedy, MA, RRT, RCP
Program Director
Respiratory Therapy Program
University of Hartford
West Hartford, Connecticut

S. Lee King, MS, RRT
Chairman
Department of Respiratory Care
Pearl River College
Hattiesburg, Massachusetts

Michael R. McCumber, EdD, RRT
Program Director
Department of Respiratory Therapy
Daytona Beach Community College
Daytona Beach, Florida

Michael McDonald, BS, RRT
Regional Vice President
Pediatric Services of America, Inc.
Denver, Colorado

Robert L. Wilkins, PhD, RRT
Professor and Chair
Department of Cardiopulmonary
  Sciences
School of Allied Health Professions
Loma Linda University
Loma Linda, California

Contents

chapter 1

The Rationale for Respiratory Home Care

Patrick J. Dunne, MEd, RRT
Susan L. McInturff, RCP, RRT

Historical Perspective

Patients have been receiving home care services in the United States for more than 100 years; in fact, home health care can trace its origins to 1893. Two nurses, Lillian Wald and Mary Brewster, saw the advantages of home health services over institutionalized care and from their vision the Visiting Nurses Association (VNA) was formed.[1] Throughout the first half of the century, home health care provided nursing and social services primarily to the economically disadvantaged and the homebound.

Dr. E.M. Bluestone established the first hospital-based home health care department in 1947 in New York City.[1] Bluestone believed that hospitals had a social responsibility to care for patients not only while they were hospitalized but after they left the facility as well. Bluestone envisioned what could be considered "continuum of care" in today's terminology.

Home health care has expanded since 1947, and today nearly every hospital has either a home health care department or an established relationship with a community-based provider of such services. Patients no longer must be indigent or homebound to be eligible for home care services, and home health care now includes not only nursing and social services but other disciplines as well. Physical, occupational, speech, and nutritional therapy as well as respiratory care services are now routinely provided to the home health patient.

The Current Climate of Home Health Care

The US Department of Commerce has identified home health care as the fastest-growing segment of the health care industry.[2] This trend is not surprising, considering that the traditional method of providing health care, that is, in the acute care facility, is also the most expensive method of providing health care.[3]

In 1995 health care expenditures amounted to more than $1 trillion and consumed more than 14 percent of the US gross domestic product (GDP)[4]; the GDP is projected to rise to 16 percent by the year 2000,[5] and this amount continues to escalate. As health care costs continue to rise, health insurance companies try to identify ways to reduce these expenditures, the most obvious being to provide care in less costly locations. Home health care has repeatedly been shown to be the least expensive way to provide health care.[2]

The Benefits of Home Care

As skyrocketing health care costs have turned our focus to reducing health care expenditures, a major benefit becomes apparent: Patients can be treated at home at a much lower cost than in the acute care facility. From the patient's point of view, home care fosters a level of independence and dignity and can reduce the incidence of rehospitalization. In addition, home health care:

- Decreases the hospital length of stay
- Reduces rehospitalizations
- Enhances patients' ability to independently manage their care
- Allows for emergent problems to be addressed
- Allows for monitoring the patient's response to treatment
- Helps improve the patient's quality of life
- Allows technology-dependent patients to go home rather than remain institutionalized for the remainder of their lives
- Reduces overall expenditures

Home care also benefits the respiratory care practitioner (RCP). Home care RCPs become better acquainted and establish relationships with their patients in a way that is not possible in the acute care facility. Because home care patients frequently are seen on a long-term basis, the RCP can establish a relationship with the patient, thereby viewing him or her as a person, not as a diagnosis. RCPs providing home care also develop heightened skills in assessment and decision making, because other providers are often unavailable to ask for help or an instant opinion. Home care RCPs experience a great deal of satisfaction from being instrumental in assisting the patient to go home and in helping to promote an enhanced quality of life within the confines of the disease state. Patients and their families are also very grateful for the help the home care RCP provides.

Candidates for Home Care

It is estimated that 44 percent of all patients discharged from the hospital require posthospital medical or nursing care that cannot be provided by family.[6] It is also estimated that 20 percent of patients over the age of 65 years have functional and physical problems that impair their ability to perform the essential activities of daily living.[6]

The older population, persons 65 years or more, represented 12.4 percent (31 million) of the total population in the United States in 1989 and is expected to double to almost 69 million by the year 2050.[7] The number of people aged 85 years or older is expected to be seven times larger by 2050. If one considers how many of these people will be functionally or physically impaired to the degree that they require home care, it is no wonder that this specialty area of practice is growing so rapidly.

When one looks at factors other than age and functional impairment, it becomes apparent that not just the elderly are candidates for home care. Chronic obstructive pulmonary disease (COPD) and its related conditions are ranked as the fifth leading cause of death in the United States.[8] The incidence of chronic asthma increased by 29 percent from 1980 to 1987 and shows no sign of slowing.[9] It is estimated that as many as 40 million Americans may be chronically ill with sleep-related disorders, and an additional 20 to 30 million people are experiencing intermittent sleep-related problems.[10] The number of patients diagnosed with human immunodeficiency virus (HIV) and acquired immunodeficiency syndrome (AIDS) and other community-acquired illnesses is increasing daily. Patients with these types of chronic medical problems require long-term treatment that is now being administered increasingly in the home.

The primary candidate for home care is the patient who is being discharged from the hospital while still requiring medical treatment. Patients are being discharged much earlier in the course of their treatment or may

ADL~ activities for daily living

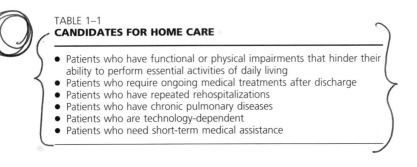

TABLE 1–1
CANDIDATES FOR HOME CARE

- Patients who have functional or physical impairments that hinder their ability to perform essential activities of daily living
- Patients who require ongoing medical treatments after discharge
- Patients who have repeated rehospitalizations
- Patients who have chronic pulmonary diseases
- Patients who are technology-dependent
- Patients who need short-term medical assistance

be technology-dependent (i.e., the tracheostomy patient, the patient on a home ventilator), yet still want to go home. These patients are no longer kept in the acute care setting or nursing home if it is at all possible to send them home.

Table 1–1 reviews the candidates for respiratory home care.

The Role of the Respiratory Care Practitioner

The focus in health care is shifting away from the acute care facility to alternate sites, and RCPs are looking to these sites for employment. This trend is certainly being driven to a large degree by hospital downsizing and the cross-training of other hospital employees to perform respiratory care services. RCPs who are finding fewer jobs available in the acute care setting are finding them in alternate sites such as subacute and home care.

Not every RCP is suited to performing respiratory home care. RCPs who cannot imagine life without the excitement of the intensive care unit or emergency room may not appreciate the challenges of home care. Others may not feel comfortable teaching a patient how to use a piece of equipment that is not related to respiratory care, such as a walker or an enteral pump. Still others will not like the driving required to deliver home care. It takes a very special clinician with a defined set of skills and expertise to successfully work in the home care arena.

Home Medical and Respiratory Therapy Equipment Services

Home health care is defined as "the provision of services and equipment to patients in the home for the purposes of restoring and maintaining their maximal level of comfort, function, and health."[11] The majority of RCPs practicing home care are employed by providers of home medical and respiratory therapy equipment (HME/RT) services.

HME/RT providers arrange for the selection, delivery, setup, use, and ongoing maintenance of medically necessary equipment in the home.

HME – based on medical necessity

HME/RT companies employ RCPs to perform these services when respiratory-related equipment is ordered for a patient. The RCP teaches the patient to properly use and maintain the equipment in accordance with the physician's prescription. The RCP also makes an initial home visit to assess the patient and caregivers, evaluate the home environment, and train any caregivers about the prescribed equipment.

One might assume that, after the respiratory equipment is set up, the RCP is finished working with the patient. This is not the case, however. Once the initial visit is made and the equipment is set up, the RCP develops an individualized plan of care/service for the patient and determines a follow-up schedule. Follow-up allows for telephone calls or home visits as often as necessary, physical assessments as approved by the physician in the plan of care/service, and reeducation as necessary. The RCP modifies and updates the plan of care/service based on the status of the patient. Follow-up continues until the therapy is discontinued or until all of the goals in the individualized plan have been met and the patient is capable of managing his or her own care.

Not all RCPs practicing home care are employed by HME/RT companies. Home health agencies that employ nurses and other allied health professionals to provide intermittent skilled home visits occasionally have an RCP on staff to assist with pulmonary patients, although this is fairly unusual. Home health agencies are reimbursed by Medicare and other insurance companies for home visits made by nurses; physical, occupational, and speech therapists; social workers; and home health aides. Regrettably, home health agencies are not typically reimbursed for home visits provided by the RCP, because most insurance carriers follow Medicare's rules and guidelines, and home visits by an RCP are not currently a benefit of the Medicare program. However, the costs associated with having an RCP employed by a home health agency are considered part of that agency's overhead and, thus, an allowed expense on the annual cost report. For this reason few home health agencies use an RCP as part of their staff. Other RCPs may make home visits for hospitals or physicians' offices but, again, these visits are not reimbursed by most insurance carriers, including Medicare.

HME/RT providers do not receive reimbursement for RCP home visits, either. HME/RT providers see the necessity of having RCPs on staff to provide the professional services that go along with providing medical equipment. Referral sources expect companies to have an RCP on staff before they will refer patients, and HME/RT companies can provide a greater variety of home medical equipment when they have an RCP on staff.

Requisite Skills

Not every RCP is suited to working in a neonatal intensive care unit or in a smoking cessation program or to managing a respiratory care department.

TABLE 1–2

QUALIFICATIONS OF THE HOME CARE RESPIRATORY CARE PRACTITIONER

The ideal home care RCP:

- Must be a graduate of a respiratory therapy program accredited by the Commission on Accreditation for Allied Health Educational Programs (CAAHEP)
- Must be credentialed by the National Board for Respiratory Care (NBRC)
- Must hold a current license or certification in the state in which they seek employment (where applicable)
- Must have at least 1 year of acute care clinical experience following graduation
- Should have experience working with both pediatric and geriatric patients
- Must be able to perform all types of respiratory therapy modalities
- Must have excellent communication skills at all levels (physicians, other health professionals, lay persons, children)
- Must have good assessment skills.
- Must be able to teach others
- Must be able to work unsupervised
- Must possess good decision-making skills
- Must be able to manage time carefully
- Must be capable of organizing information and presenting in-services
- Must possess a valid driver's license
- Must have adequate automobile insurance
- Must be comfortable with driving a good deal
- Must be willing to participate in community-based organizations (Chamber of Commerce, Lung Association, etc.)
- being on call after hours
- CPR

Each specialty area of practice requires the RCP to possess certain skills. This is true for home care as well. Not every RCP has what it takes to be a home care clinician. The home care RCP must possess top-level skills such as assessment, decision making, patient education, and time management. Table 1–2 lists the qualifications of a home care RCP.

Assessment

The ability to assess many different aspects of the patient is probably the most important skill for a home care RCP to possess. Assessment of the patient in the acute care setting is fairly narrow in scope: The RCP makes a limited physical assessment of the patient's pulmonary status. Also, the hospital-based RCP uses many diagnostic tools to assist in the evaluation of the patient's pulmonary status.

The RCP's assessment of the home care patient could include a complete physical evaluation as well as a comprehensive interview to determine the patient's medical history. The RCP also evaluates the patient's physical environment and equipment needs. An assessment of any caregivers, including their capabilities and willingness to provide care, is also performed by the home care RCP. Identification of any psychosocial issues that might affect the patient's care is part of the RCP's assessment, as well. Although the acute care RCP uses many diagnostic tools in making assessments, the home care RCP uses only the most basic: a stethoscope, a blood pressure cuff, and possibly an oximeter.

The RCP must have a keen eye and know what to look for and where to look when assessing the home care patient. The RCP must understand the parameters that are assessed, such as the significance of pitting edema, conditions affecting a blood pressure or oximeter reading, or an improperly grounded electrical outlet's effect on the patient's use of his or her respiratory therapy equipment. A thorough assessment gives the RCP a baseline from which to compare the patient at subsequent visits, allowing the RCP to identify emergent problems.

Decision Making

Another important skill the home care RCP must possess is that of decision making. The home care RCP must make decisions regarding the patient's treatment in terms of the physician's prescription, while taking into account all the information that was gathered during the patient assessment. The RCP often has to decide on appropriate types of equipment based on the patient's functional or physical limitations. For example, a patient with poor vision may require an oxygen system with a flow controller that "clicks" at each flow setting, allowing the patient to count the number of clicks to set the flow controller correctly. The RCP may decide that the patient with severe arthritis in the hands will not be able to turn on a portable E tank with a cylinder key and that another type of portable oxygen system will be needed to meet the patient's needs.

The RCP must make decisions about the patient's treatment based on psychosocial issues. The patient who lives alone and cannot measure the medications for nebulizer treatments may require a change to unit dose medications. The RCP may determine that the patient's spouse is not willing to learn to suction the patient and so must identify and train another caregiver. The RCP may even have to decide that emergency medical treatment is indicated in a patient who has not specified any advance directives.

The RCP must be able to make decisions without the support and expertise of other RCPs. Home care RCPs generally work alone, and, although more than one RCP may be working for the HME/RT provider, they are all usually seeing their own patients and are not easily available to one another during the course of the day. The home care RCP consults with the physician, the home health nurse (if the patient is being followed by a home health agency), and other members of the patient's home care team for assistance, however.

Many institutions use therapist-driven protocols or care mapping to help the RCP in decision making. These "if this, then that" protocols are helpful in guiding the clinician along the right course. Regrettably, there is a scarcity of such tools in home care. Clinical practice guidelines and individual

HME/RT company policies and procedures are the only decision-making tools available to the home care RCP at this time.

Patient Education

The home care RCP spends a good deal of time teaching the patient and any caregivers about the safe and effective use of many different types of home medical equipment. The RCP also instructs the patient and caregivers about pulmonary diseases, symptom recognition and management, and infection control. Because of this educational role, the RCP must be able to convey information and instructions to the patient and caregivers in an understandable way and to reinstruct the patient as necessary.

The home care RCP is attempting to teach a lay person to use technical equipment and perform complex medical procedures that are traditionally performed by a professional in a controlled setting. Learning is a very individualized process, and no one teaching method will work for everyone. Some people learn best through visual aids such as videotapes, pictures, and written instructions. Others learn best with auditory aids such as lectures or audiotapes. Still others learn by doing.

All three methods can be helpful when educating the patient and the caregivers. The home care RCP might demonstrate the use of the equipment, ask for a return demonstration, and leave the patient with written materials outlining the use of the equipment. Training periods should be limited in time and the RCP should provide only the information needed to manage the equipment or the patient's care. Lecturing patients about the history of oxygen therapy will do little but confuse them. Explaining all the methods of suctioning to a patient is not particularly useful when the patient requires only oral suctioning. In addition, the instructions should be given by the same RCP each time to avoid conflicting instructions, which also might confuse the patient.

The RCP must give instructions in terms (and language, if the patient is non–English speaking) each patient or caregiver can understand. The RCP should avoid using technical terms except when necessary. If the patient refers to the medication nebulizer as a "peace pipe," the RCP should demonstrate how to put the medication into the peace pipe. It may be easier for the caregiver to refer to the ventilator circuit as the "blue hoses." It is often easier for the RCP to understand the patient's or caregiver's meaning than the opposite. Again, printed instructions with pictures are very helpful; if the patient or caregivers are non–English speaking, the printed materials may have to be translated.

The home care RCP may also be asked to provide in-service education for other health care professionals or patient support groups. These in-services frequently concern a specific topic of home respiratory care, like home oxygen therapy. They may also relate to a specific respiratory care procedure, like tracheostomy care or suctioning. The RCP must be capable of organizing information for presentation and must feel comfortable talking to groups and answering questions.

Time Management

The ability to manage time is a very important skill for the home care RCP. The RCP's goal each day is to spend as much time as possible on patient care. Many providers establish quotas of patients the RCP must see in a day to assist the RCP in time management.

Decision making plays a key role in time management. The RCP must establish which patients need home visits and determine their geographical locations. Proper routing of home visits allows for minimal driving time and maximal patient care time. It is more time-efficient to schedule home visits with patients who live in a common geographical area. If the RCP's goal is to return to the office at the end of the day, it would be ideal to schedule the most remote patient first and then work back toward the office with each successive visit.

Good assessment skills and decision making will also identify patients who may not require home visits but instead can be followed by telephone calls. A home visit to a stable patient who has met all prescribed goals amounts to nothing more than a social call and demonstrates poor time management. This is important because the HME/RT company pays the RCP to make home visits for which the company receives no reimbursement. Each patient must be thoroughly assessed, with follow-up determined by their clinical needs, not a fixed, routine schedule. A patient should not be seen every 90 days just because he or she has a certain piece of equipment; ideally, the patient should be followed only as frequently as clinical needs dictate.

Other Requirements

Many HME/RT providers require that the RCP have at least 1 year of acute care experience before he or she can be hired for home care. This acute care experience is very valuable, as it allows the RCP time to develop skills in assessment and decision making. The acute care experience also gives the RCP time to perform many of the respiratory care procedures as well as to gain confidence in his or her ability to perform these procedures in a supervised setting. Prior experience in both pediatric and geriatric pulmonary medicine is also extremely helpful, as these are the patient populations seen most often in the home care setting.

Reputable HME/RT companies will hire only licensed RCPs (where licensure is applicable) to perform respiratory care procedures and follow up on their clinical respiratory patients. Some companies also require the

RCP to possess either a certification (Certified Respiratory Therapy Technician [CRTT]) or a registry credential (Registered Respiratory Therapist [RRT]).

Most HME/RT companies require a valid driver's license and proof of a safe driving record, particularly if the company provides the RCP with a vehicle. If the RCP uses his or her own car, the company may require proof of adequate automobile insurance. RCPs going into home care for the first time must be aware of the amount of driving required, which is especially increased if the RCP is responsible for a large territory. The RCP must be prepared to drive in varied weather conditions and must be comfortable with driving in remote areas as well as in bumper-to-bumper traffic.

Home care RCPs are often required to be on call for their employer. Most HME/RT companies offer 24-hour service, necessitating the RCP to be available to set up respiratory equipment or solve clinical problems after normal business hours and on weekends. The RCP must be prepared to receive a call in the middle of the night to set up a suction machine or troubleshoot a home ventilator. On-call policies vary greatly from company to company; a common schedule is to be on call for 1 week at a time.

HME/RT providers may or may not require the RCP to possess current certification in cardiopulmonary resuscitation (CPR). Most companies do not offer CPR as a service but will respect the clinician's decision to perform it if he or she thinks it is required.

Management of Information

RCPs are required to document everything they do, regardless of the site of care. The home care RCP also documents everything from home visits to follow-up telephone calls, to route sheets, to mileage logs.

Clinical documentation, or patient charting, is carried out for any patient for whom the RCP conducts any type of follow-up. The format for this documentation varies from company to company. The RCP may carry out clinical documentation on computer, by special checklists and "fill-in-the-blank" charting forms, or even by narrative.

The home care RCP is required to document all patient instruction that is given during the home visit, and patients are asked to sign a document stating that they received the instruction. The initial home visit assessments, patient history, and the plan of care/service are also documented. Results of telephone consultations and even directions to the patient's home should be recorded in the patient's clinical chart.

Equipment maintenance records are also completed by the home care RCP. Clear and accurate records are necessary regarding cleaning, routine and preventive maintenance, and repair history of every piece of respiratory equipment used. Some equipment records for home respiratory equipment may be kept by the employee responsible for repair and maintenance for an HME company. RCPs may be responsible for keeping calibration and checkout records on equipment that they use, clean, and service, such as oxygen analyzers, oximeters, ventilators, and apnea monitors.

SUMMARY

The home care RCP plays a very important role in the overall care of the patient who has been transferred to home with continuing care needs. The home care RCP evaluates the patient, selects the appropriate equipment based on the physician's prescription, and instructs the patient and caregivers in safe and effective use of the equipment. The RCP evaluates the home environment to identify any hazards or impediments to the care of the patient. Home care RCPs also evaluate the patient and caregivers to determine their ability to manage the equipment and care for the patient.

Once the evaluations are completed, the RCP develops an individualized plan of care/service to establish goals for the patient and to determine an appropriate follow-up schedule. During each follow-up visit, the RCP reassesses the patient to determine whether the goals have been met and to evaluate the outcomes. The RCP will reinstruct, modify, or set new goals based on the patient's progress. The primary goal is to encourage the patient's own management of his or her care, a concept often referred to as "collaborative self-care."[12]

It may seem as though the home care RCP must function as part nurse, part social worker, part teacher, and part mechanic. Actually, this is exactly what the well-rounded home care therapist is. Functioning in all these ways allows the home care RCP to help the patient maintain the best possible quality of life, to provide quality care to the patient in the most cost-efficient manner, and, it is to be hoped, to reduce the incidence of future hospitalizations.

REFERENCES

1. Foreman, S: Hospital-based home care: Looking forward to the future. The Remington report. Remington Group, Laguna Niguel, CA, Oct/Nov 1993:25.
2. The case for home care. US News and World Report, April 26, 1993:71.
3. Dunne, PJ: Demographics and financial impact of home respiratory care. Respiratory Care 4:309, 1994.
4. Health Care Prognosis. Business Week, April 7, 1997, p 8.
5. Stoller, TF: What is driving change in health care delivery today? Respiratory Care 42:20, 1997.
6. Home Care Advisory Panel: Guidelines for the Medical Management of the Home Care Patient. American Medical Association, Chicago, 1992.
7. US General Accounting Office: Long-term care: Projected needs of the aging baby boom generation. GAO/HRD 91:86,1991.

8. Centers for Disease Control: Monthly vital statistics report. National Center for Health Statistics, US Department of Health and Human Services, Public Health Service, Bethesda, MD, Aug 28, 1991.

9. National Heart, Lung, and Blood Institute: Guidelines for the Diagnosis and Management of Asthma. National Institutes of Health, US Department of Health and Human Services, Public Health Service, Bethesda, MD, Aug 1991.

10. Dement, WC: Executive Summary and Executive Report, Vol I: The National Commission on Sleep Disorders Research, US Government Printing Office, Washington, DC, Jan 1993.

11. Council on Scientific Affairs: Home care in the 1990's. JAMA 9:1241, 1990.

12. Make, BJ et al: Mechanical ventilation beyond the critical care unit: Report of a consensus conference of the American College of Chest Physicians. Chest 1997, in press.

chapter 2

The Home Visit

Patrick J. Dunne, MEd, RRT
Susan L. McInturff, RCP, RRT

The RCP's visit to the home is a principal aspect of the provision of home respiratory care. It is not as simple as the home care RCP's delivering a piece of respiratory therapy equipment to the patient's home after a physician orders it. Rather, it is part of a series of events that begin when the need for home respiratory care is first identified.

Home respiratory care involves patient selection and discharge planning. It also involves assessment, education, and training. Observation, planning, and decision making are skills the home care RCP uses with each and every patient. Many of these elements take place during the home visit.

This chapter describes the various components of the respiratory home care visit. The elements of the initial home visit and the development of a plan of care/service are discussed in detail. The process of follow-up visits, patient education and training, and patient discharge from home respiratory care services is also reviewed.

The Referral

The provision of respiratory home care services actually begins when the home medical and respiratory therapy equipment (HME/RT) provider is contacted by the physician, hospital discharge planner, home health nurse, or other entity to order the home respiratory therapy equipment. This is known as the *referral.*

Patients are referred to providers of HME/RT because of their need to have their chronic medical conditions treated at home. Some patients are identified while still in the hospital as needing respiratory home care, and the HME/RT company is contacted to provide equipment and services when the patient is discharged to home. This is particularly true today, as patients are being discharged from the hospital "quicker and sicker" and require continued medical treatment.[1]

Other patients may be identified as candidates for respiratory home care during a visit to their physician's office or medical clinic or during participation in an outpatient pulmonary or cardiac rehabilitation program. The visiting nurse may identify a patient as a candidate for respiratory home care during a home health visit.

Once the need is identified, the physician will determine which respiratory home care services are indicated, such as home oxygen or aerosol therapy, continuous nasal positive airway pressure therapy, or even long-term mechanical ventilation. At this point, contact is made with the HME/RT provider, usually in the form of a telephone call from the referral source. This sets the "admission to service" process in motion.

The Discharge Plan

It was stated earlier that hospitalized patients are frequently referred to an HME/RT provider for their home care services. Unfortunately, this referral most often occurs just as the patient is about to go home. In many instances, this last-minute arrangement is sufficient; for patients requiring respiratory therapy equipment, however, it is not always the ideal method of obtaining home care.

The ideal method is the use of a discharge planning process. This is a comprehensive plan that identifies, well before the last minute, the patient's needs and appraises issues such as financial resources, reimbursement, caregivers and their abilities, and medical equipment needs.[2,3] Ideally, this plan

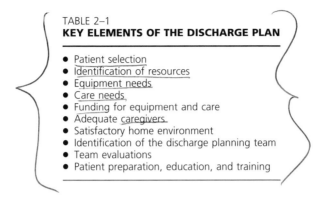

TABLE 2–1
KEY ELEMENTS OF THE DISCHARGE PLAN

- Patient selection
- Identification of resources
- Equipment needs
- Care needs
- Funding for equipment and care
- Adequate caregivers
- Satisfactory home environment
- Identification of the discharge planning team
- Team evaluations
- Patient preparation, education, and training

is developed prior to imminent discharge to allow time for problems to be resolved. Table 2–1 lists the key elements of a meaningful discharge plan.

The complexity of the discharge plan is relative to the patient's medical condition and medical equipment needs as well as the number of problems or other issues found during the evaluation process. For example, the patient who requires compressor-nebulizer therapy, has insurance coverage for it, and is capable of complete medical self-management will not require the same level of discharge planning as a patient going home on long-term invasive mechanical ventilation. However, failure to thoroughly evaluate a compressor-nebulizer patient and his or her home situation could result in serious consequences if the patient were unable to measure medications properly, could not afford the medications, or lived in a trailer without electricity. This is precisely the reason for having a discharge plan for each patient, regardless of the apparent simplicity of his or her needs.

The discharge planning process should be initiated as early as possible in the acute care setting.[2,3] This early planning falls in line with the desire to shorten the patient's acute hospital stay. The rule now is to start planning for discharge as soon as the patient is admitted into the hospital, which allows more time to identify problems and correct them or to alter the plan before the patient is actually discharged. If a patient cannot afford medications for a compressor-nebulizer, early problem identification allows time to explore alternative sources of funding or to alter the therapy regimen to make it more feasible for the patient.

The discharge planning process is frequently coordinated by a single person. Discharge planners are often nurses or medical social workers with a limited background in respiratory care. However, the discharge planner may also be an RCP on staff at the hospital. The discharge planner coordinates the efforts of a team of health care professionals, both hospital- and home care–based. Table 2–2 lists the health care professionals that may be a part of the discharge planning team. These team members evaluate the patient, develop and implement the discharge plan, and provide the home care

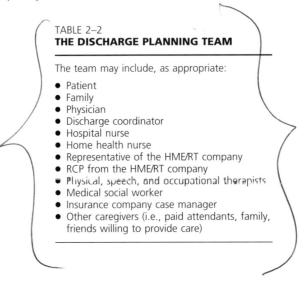

TABLE 2–2
THE DISCHARGE PLANNING TEAM

The team may include, as appropriate:

- Patient
- Family
- Physician
- Discharge coordinator
- Hospital nurse
- Home health nurse
- Representative of the HME/RT company
- RCP from the HME/RT company
- Physical, speech, and occupational therapists
- Medical social worker
- Insurance company case manager
- Other caregivers (i.e., paid attendants, family, friends willing to provide care)

services. Which professionals are used depends on the complexity of the plan and the needs of the patient.

Development of the discharge plan is based on the physician's discharge orders. These orders specify the types of therapy and services intended for the patient to use at home. The discharge planner takes the physician's order and identifies the team members needed to prepare the patient to receive the appropriate care at home.

Preparing the Patient for Discharge

Preparing the patient for discharge includes evaluation of the patient's medical condition. Examination or tests needed to justify third-party reimbursement of any medical equipment should be performed. For example, blood gases or oxygen saturation by pulse oximetry may be needed to justify home oxygen therapy, a polysomnogram may be needed to justify continuous positive airway pressure (CPAP) therapy, or a pneumogram may be needed to justify an apnea monitor. The medical evaluation should also identify the patient's actual treatment needs, such as oxygen liter flow at rest, with activities (and which activities), and during sleep.

Evaluating the Patient

The predischarge evaluation should also identify any functional or physical limitations the patient may have that could affect the ability to manage his or her own care, such as vision problems that would hinder the patient's capacity to correctly adjust the flowmeter on an oxygen system. Evaluating the patient's functional and physical impairments will also help identify the need for outside assistance such as home nursing or respiratory care services.

Evaluating the Caregivers — Support System

Discharge preparations should also include the identification and evaluation of family members and other caregivers the patient may need if the patient is unable to manage his or her own care. These caregivers must be assessed to determine their willingness to provide care, their capabilities, and their ability to learn the required skills. The patient's discharge plan may require alteration if the needed caregivers are not available.

Evaluating the Home Environment

The patient's home environment should be evaluated before discharge whenever possible. This evaluation is especially important when multiple pieces of medical equipment may be required. The home assessment is most frequently made during the home care RCP's initial visit, but in complex cases it is desirable to evaluate the home for any fire, safety, or health hazards before sending the patient home if the home could prove to be an unsuitable environment. An evaluation of the patient's physical environment should *always* be made for those patients requiring home mechanical ventilation at discharge.[2,4]

Reimbursement

The discharge plan should also include a determination of whether reimbursement for ordered equipment and related care/service will be covered by the patient's medical insurance. The home care RCP should never assume that an insurance company will pay for something just because the physician orders it; rather, third-party payers require medical justification before they will authorize payment. Also, the RCP should never assume that the patient will want the equipment just because the physician orders it, particularly if it is not covered by insurance. Many patients will decline equipment or therapy if they have to pay for it themselves. It is preferable to make these determinations before any equipment is actually placed in the home.

Education and Training

Another important part of the discharge planning process in which the home care RCP plays a role is that of patient and caregiver educator. The amount of education and training required to prepare the patient for discharge is largely dependent on two critical factors: (1) the type of respiratory care needed by the patient and (2) the ability and willingness of the patient to assume responsibility for collaborative self-care. The patient who requires a compressor-nebulizer may need instruction only on the frequency of treatments, a review of medications used in the nebulizer, and the infection control procedures. The patient with a tracheostomy tube will require more extensive training to ensure the patient's or caregivers' abilities to manage suctioning, tracheostomy tube care, and other required procedures.

As part of the discharge planning team, the RCP will assist with patient education and training during the discharge planning process. Some types of home respiratory therapy equipment such as mechanical ventilators, suction machines, and apnea monitors are brought into the hospital and put into use on the patient to better familiarize the patient and any caregivers with the equipment's operation. The hospital-based RCP assisting with teaching should be familiar with the home medical equipment that is brought into the hospital as well as with procedures such as suctioning, tracheostomy care, and cleaning and disinfection as performed in the home care setting. This is extremely important in preventing the patient and caregivers from receiving conflicting instructions from hospital- and home care–based RCPs.

During the predischarge training process, patients should be instructed to perform all care procedures themselves whenever possible. Training sessions should (1) be kept short, (2) be limited in scope, (3) be geared to the specific needs of the patient, and (4) encourage interaction. Studies have shown that patients and caregivers rate emergency, physical, and safety skills as being most important for them to learn. Knowledge of lung disease processes was rated as being the least important.[5,6] The RCP must also remember that the patient may be learning other care procedures during the predischarge training and should take care not to overwhelm the patient with too much information and training at one time.

Each person learns differently and at a different pace, so interaction should be encouraged to determine the information being retained. It may be helpful to use videotaped presentations of care procedures or to have printed instructions containing the necessary information that the learner can review as needed. Having the patient and caregivers observe the procedures as the RCP performs them is a helpful method of training. The RCP should provide step-by-step explanations of the procedure that is being performed, the way each step is tolerated by the patient, signs and symptoms to watch for, and steps to take in the event of an emergency during the procedure. Once it has been determined that the patient and caregivers understand how to perform a procedure, they should be asked to perform it with the RCP observing. Retraining should take place as indicated by the patient's or caregivers' performance. The patient and caregivers should be encouraged to perform all procedures as often as possible while the patient is still in the hospital so as to build confidence in their ability to manage the required care.

Admission to Service

Use of a discharge plan better prepares the patient for going home. Part of the discharge plan will be the referral to the HME/RT provider. Once the

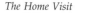

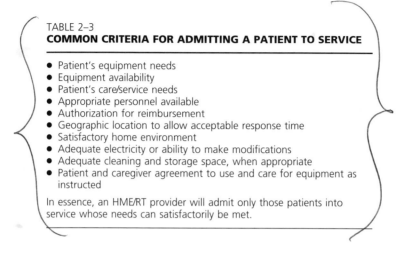

TABLE 2–3
COMMON CRITERIA FOR ADMITTING A PATIENT TO SERVICE

- Patient's equipment needs
- Equipment availability
- Patient's care/service needs
- Appropriate personnel available
- Authorization for reimbursement
- Geographic location to allow acceptable response time
- Satisfactory home environment
- Adequate electricity or ability to make modifications
- Adequate cleaning and storage space, when appropriate
- Patient and caregiver agreement to use and care for equipment as instructed

In essence, an HME/RT provider will admit only those patients into service whose needs can satisfactorily be met.

referral is made, the HME/RT provider will determine whether the patient can be admitted to service. "Admission to service" means that the company has the resources to provide the equipment and services necessary for the patient's care and that the company therefore accepts that responsibility.

Each company's acceptance criteria are different. Some companies provide only equipment management services and do not provide clinical respiratory services. A company that does not provide clinical respiratory services would not be capable of accepting a home ventilator patient. Further, a company that provides clinical respiratory services may not be able to accept a baby requiring phototherapy for hyperbilirubinemia as a patient if the company has no appropriately trained RCPs. Some companies may not accept patients with certain types of medical insurance. Most companies do not accept patients outside of the geographical area that they service.

Generally speaking, a company will admit a patient to service only if the company can meet the needs of that patient. Table 2–3 reviews common acceptance criteria. Once the patient is accepted into service, the home care RCP begins work in earnest.

The Initial Home Visit

observational only
usually 24–48 hrs so pt can ask questions

The purpose of the initial home visit is to evaluate the patient, including his or her physical environment and needs as they relate to the physician's prescription, and to establish a plan to meet these needs. If the home care RCP is included as part of the discharge planning team, much of this legwork will have already been completed. It happens much more frequently, however, that the patient has had very limited discharge planning and that the RCP will have had no contact with the patient prior to discharge.

Scheduling

Upon receiving the referral to provide home respiratory therapy services, the home care RCP makes initial telephone contact with the patient. Depending on the type of equipment that has been prescribed, the actual equipment setup may be carried out by other HME/RT personnel. Most HME/RT providers have trained delivery technicians who set up not only durable medical equipment (DME) such as hospital beds and wheelchairs but also oxygen therapy equipment. Other categories of equipment, such as apnea monitors, CPAP devices, and mechanical ventilators are best set up by the RCP. If a delivery technician sets up the equipment, the RCP will schedule the initial home visit within the first 24 to 48 hours, depending on company policy. If the RCP sets up the equipment, that time is also used to perform the components of the initial visit.

The home care RCP's day is usually spent seeing both new and ongoing patients. Some companies have quotas of patients the RCP must try to see in one day, making scheduling an important skill for the home care RCP. Home care RCPs often route their home visits within a specific geographical area to use time most efficiently. Careful routing allows for minimal driving time and maximal time for patient care. Figure 2–1 outlines a sample daily schedule for the home care RCP.

Coordinating with Other Services

Patients requiring respiratory home care services will often have other home care professionals following them, such as home health nurses, physical and occupational therapists, and medical social workers. The home care RCP should attempt to coordinate his or her services with those of the other professionals to present a team approach to the care of the patient.

Each professional will bring a different perspective to the team that can enhance the overall plan of service/care for a patient. It may be useful for the home care RCP and home health nurse to schedule a joint visit to assess the patient. This visit allows the home health nurse to have a clearer understanding of the patient's respiratory therapy needs and to better reinforce them. It also helps the home care RCP to better understand the patient's overall needs and their relationship to the patient's respiratory problems. For example, during a joint visit the home health nurse and the RCP can establish use times for the patient using home oxygen. The nurse can then reinforce on subsequent visits that, yes, the patient should use the oxygen while bathing or during sleep. The home health nurse and the RCP might also establish that the diabetic patient suffers from dyspnea when his or her blood sugar is abnormal. The home care RCP can reinforce the patient's need to check blood sugar level on a glucose monitor when having unexplained dyspnea.

Daily Schedule

Therapist _____

Date _____

PATIENT NAME	LOCATION	TIME IN	TIME OUT	SERVICE	$ COLLECTED	DRIVE TIME

Start Mileage _____

End Mileage _____

Total Mileage _____

Tolls, etc. _____

Total Visit Time _____

Total Drive Time _____

Total $ Collected _____

FIGURE 2–1
Sample daily schedule sheet.

Some patients feel overwhelmed by too many visitors in their home at one time or even in one day. They may prefer separate visits by home care professionals. The patient and caregivers should be consulted before a joint home visit to ensure that they are agreeable to it.

Coordination of services also involves communication among home health care professionals. This may occur in written form by sending the other team members a copy of the home visit report, through telephone consultation, or during team conferences to map out problems and solutions. Most important is that the team be working toward a common goal. For example, if a patient has been prescribed oxygen for use 24 hours per day, the common goal would be for that patient to use the oxygen continuously. If one team member is encouraging the patient to use the oxygen most of the time but another team member tells the patient it is acceptable to discontinue oxygen to go out to the mailbox or to run a few errands, the common goal of compliance will be compromised. If the home care RCP has evaluated an oxygen patient and has determined that the patient indeed desaturates when oxygen is interrupted, that home care RCP can make the other team members aware of this fact so that no one recommends that the patient be weaned or that oxygen use be otherwise interrupted.

The Initial Assessment ⟶ med profile, environ safety

The first home visit is very important in the overall care of the patient because of all the information that is collected at this time. This information helps the home care RCP to make decisions regarding the most appropriate equipment for the patient, care or service plan structure, and type of follow-up schedule.

The Patient Interview

The home care RCP will perform a patient and caregiver interview to ascertain the patient's medical history and symptom profile.[7,8] This interview is comprehensive and will help identify medical, familial, psychosocial, and cultural issues that may have an impact on a patient's care. The interview should also establish whether the patient is going to manage his or her own care; identify the caregivers, if needed; and determine whether the caregivers are willing and able to perform the necessary care.

Assessment of Functional and Physical Impairments

Patients receiving respiratory home care should also be evaluated for functional or physical limitations.[1,7,8] Poor vision, poor hand strength, and other physical impairments can make it difficult for a patient to operate medical devices such as oxygen regulators. Hearing disabilities can make

TABLE 2–4
**FUNCTIONAL AND PHYSICAL LIMITATIONS TO
EVALUATE DURING THE INITIAL ASSESSMENT**

- Are you able to walk unaided? Are you able to walk without shortness of breath? Are you able to climb stairs? Do you need to use a walker, cane, or other walking aid? Do you have any weakness, arthritis, or swelling in your feet, ankles, or legs?
- Do you have arthritis in your hands? Are you able to close your hands and make a fist? Are you unable to do any activities because of problems with your hands? Are your hands shaky? Are you able to lift lightweight objects?
- Do you have any hearing or vision problems? Can you read your medicine containers easily? Can you read the gauges, flowmeters, or other indicators on your home medical equipment? Are you able to hear the alarms made by the equipment? Can you hear your telephone when it rings?
- Are you able to shower or bathe without assistance? Are you able to put on your clothes without assistance? Are you exhausted or short of breath after bathing or dressing?
- Are you able to make your bed without help? Who does your cleaning and laundry?
- Are you able to cook for yourself? Do you do your own shopping? How many meals do you eat per day? How much water do you drink each day?
- Does your breathing problem limit your lifestyle at all? Are you limited in any way by shortness of breath?
- Do you feel your oxygen equipment limits you in any way?
- Have you ever been taught energy conservation techniques or special breathing techniques?
- Are you able to remember to take your medications and breathing treatments?

it difficult for a patient to hear and respond to equipment alarms. Speech problems or language barriers can impair a patient's ability to communicate his or her needs. Cognitive disabilities can make equipment operation instructions difficult to comprehend. Patients with poor short-term memory may not be able to remember when or if they have taken their medicines. Poor memory can interfere with a patient's ability to refill a portable oxygen unit. Problems with ambulating, such as unsteady gait or the need for assistive devices such as a walker, cane, or wheelchair, can present challenges to the patient, such as when oxygen tubing is lying on the floor. For optimum results, this evaluation must be comprehensive. Table 2–4 lists various functional and physical impairments that should be evaluated.

Caregivers should also be evaluated for the same functional and physical limitations, which could interfere with their ability to provide care. A patient for whom nebulized medications are prescribed but who cannot self-administer the treatment may not receive the required therapy if a spouse or other caregivers have functional or physical limitations that render them unable to administer the treatment. Should the home care RCP determine that the spouse or caregiver is unable to safely operate the required medical equipment or perform the necessary care procedures, alternate caregivers must be identified and they, in turn, must be evaluated. If no other caregivers are available, the home care RCP will have to determine whether it is safe for

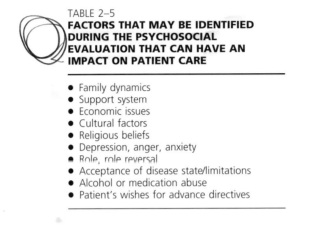

TABLE 2–5
**FACTORS THAT MAY BE IDENTIFIED
DURING THE PSYCHOSOCIAL
EVALUATION THAT CAN HAVE AN
IMPACT ON PATIENT CARE**

- Family dynamics
- Support system
- Economic issues
- Cultural factors
- Religious beliefs
- Depression, anger, anxiety
- Role, role reversal
- Acceptance of disease state/limitations
- Alcohol or medication abuse
- Patient's wishes for advance directives

the patient to receive home respiratory care and whether admission to service is appropriate.

Psychosocial Assessment

Another important aspect of the initial assessment is the psychosocial evaluation. Just as there are aspects of the patient's medical condition that can affect care, there are aspects of emotional, cultural, and familial status that can affect care as well.[8,9] Table 2–5 highlights factors that the home care RCP should evaluate during the psychosocial assessment.

Patients with chronic pulmonary conditions often exhibit signs of hopelessness or anger because of their illness.[10] The patient who is receiving home oxygen therapy for the first time may feel that the oxygen system is a "ball and chain" to which he or she will be forever tied. Patients may feel as though they can no longer leave the house or conduct life in their previous manner. Patients receiving home mechanical ventilation may express anger due to their dependency on a machine to keep them breathing and their dependency on others for even their most basic needs.

Depression is often a problem for patients with chronic pulmonary disease.[9] For many patients, depression can lead to thoughts or plans of suicide. Respiratory care training does not yet prepare the home care RCP to determine whether a patient is truly suicidal or just conveying frustration. Therefore, the home care RCP must take seriously any patient who expresses such thoughts or details a suicide plan and must contact the physician. If a medical social worker or home health nurse is involved in the patient's care, the RCP should inform him or her as well.

Cultural factors can also have an impact on a patient's home care. The male spouse who has always been the head of the household may have difficulty adjusting to the role reversal that takes place when severe chronic lung disease makes it impossible to perform even the simplest of tasks for himself. Conversely, the family in which the wife has been responsible for the domestic chores while caring for her family may find it difficult to cope when illness prevents her from performing these duties. Home care patients and their families often express dismay over the changes in their relationships with others, particularly with other family members.[10]

A patient's cultural background may call for an extended family to live together under one roof. This can be a great benefit to the patient requiring a lot of care because many potential caregivers are living in the home. It can prove to be a detriment, however, if some of those extended family members are small children or others who also require care. Space can be an issue when many family members live in a single home, particularly when the home is small. Another cultural issue that occurs with some frequency and may be an irritant to some home care RCPs is the request to remove their shoes before entering the patient's home. The RCP should always respect the patient's wishes and comply with such requests.

Assessment of the Physical Environment

The home care RCP should *always* perform an evaluation of the patient's physical environment during the initial home visit. This evaluation is an inspection of the patient's home to identify any fire, safety, or additional health hazards that could affect use of equipment or provision of care.[11]

Inspecting a patient's home can prove to be a delicate matter. The home care RCP must bear in mind that a patient's home is his or her "castle" and that everyone has a different lifestyle. A patient's view of an acceptable environment may not necessarily fit the RCP's characterization of an appropriate living environment. For example, everyone has a different idea of what constitutes a clean, orderly, and safe living environment. Although the home care RCP is assessing for hazards and impediments, patients should be asked to change their environment and lifestyle as little as possible. Table 2–6 lists important elements to evaluate in the patient's physical environment. Patients may reasonably request that certain areas of the home not be inspected if the area in question is not required for the provision of care or service.

One of the most critical conditions to inspect is a home's electrical capabilities. This is particularly true when multiple pieces of electrically powered medical equipment are going to be used, as is the case with home ventilator patients. Electrical circuits must carry enough amperage to manage the medical equipment as well as any home appliances the patient or caregiver may want to use at the same time. Consider the patient using an oxygen concentrator in the living room: There may be the oxygen concentrator, lamps, television, VCR, space heater, motorized recliner, and other appliances all on the same circuit. Depending on the amperage of that circuit, a

TABLE 2–6
ELEMENTS OF THE PHYSICAL ENVIRONMENT ASSESSMENT

- Is there adequate space in which to place the medical equipment? Is there storage space for supplies?
- Is there adequate electricity to power the equipment? Are the electrical outlets grounded? Will it be necessary to use 3- to 2-prong adapters, extension cords, or power strips?
- Are there working smoke detectors in the home? How many?
- Are there any fire extinguishers in the home? Where are they located? Are they fully charged?
- Is there a telephone in the home? Are there any extensions?
- Is there enough lighting to read the gauges and dials on the equipment or to perform care procedures?
- Are the home's walkways clear? Is there more than one exit? Is there an emergency exit plan?
- Are there any problems with cleanliness that could affect patient care?
- Is there a place to clean and disinfect equipment?
- Does the home have adequate heating and cooling equipment? Are these systems powered by electricity?
- Does the home use well water?
- Does the home have a backup generator? How frequently do power outages occur?
- Are there any identifiable safety hazards? Do the floors have throw rugs that could present a hazard for ambulating? Are there stairs the patient must navigate?

patient may trip the circuit breaker when turning on the oxygen concentrator. Given the choice of using the television or the oxygen concentrator, the patient may very likely choose the television. The patient may need to move appliances to other circuits in the home or the RCP may have to relocate the medical equipment. Multiplug power strips can be useful for plugging in several pieces of equipment, but the power strips must be high grade and in optimum working order.

The RCP may need to inspect the home's fuse or circuit box to determine how many circuits the home has and for how many amps the circuits are rated. Most homes have 15-amp circuits. The RCP should verify that fuses are in place if circuit breakers are not being used and that the fuses are the correct size. Adding up the amperage requirements of the equipment will give the RCP an idea of whether more than one circuit will be needed; the amperage is usually listed on a label on the equipment or in the specifications section of the equipment's operation manual.

The home care RCP should also determine whether the home's electrical outlets are properly grounded. Grounded outlets reduce the risk of electrical shock. Hardware stores carry simple outlet testers that plug into the electrical outlet and light up to demonstrate proper and improper grounding (Fig. 2–2). If the outlet that the medical equipment is being plugged into is not properly grounded, the patient must be informed of the increased risk of electrical shock. A 3- to 2-prong electrical adapter may be used if properly installed.

Older homes can present some special challenges. These homes may

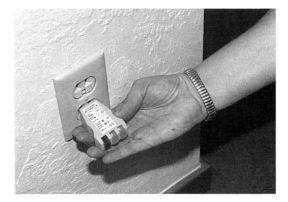

FIGURE 2–2
Home care RCP checking outlets for proper grounding.

have inadequate numbers of circuits or improper circuit breakers or fuses. It is not uncommon to find a fuse box without fuses or a penny in place of the fuse. It can be very helpful to have the home inspected by a professional electrician when there is any doubt about the home's electrical capabilities. Modifications may be necessary to use the medical equipment safely. Bear in mind, however, that this may be an expense the patient cannot afford. If the home requires modifications that the patient cannot make, the home care RCP may need to use alternate types of equipment like nonelectric oxygen equipment. Battery-powered equipment can also be used, but the patient must have a source of electricity to recharge the batteries. Depending on the equipment needed, it may not be safe to provide medical equipment to the patient in this circumstance.

The home should be evaluated to determine whether it has adequate space for the equipment and supplies the patient needs. It may be necessary for the patient to rearrange or remove furniture and other items that might interfere with access to the patient or the equipment. The home should also have enough space to keep medical devices away from heaters, fireplaces, or other sources of flame. Functioning smoke detectors should be in the home, and fire extinguishers are desirable. The RCP should recommend these safety items if the patient does not already have them installed.

The home care RCP should identify all exits, and an emergency exit route should be mapped out. Walkways should be clear, and stairways should have secure banisters. There should be adequate heating and cooling systems as well as adequate lighting. An acceptable equipment cleaning, disinfection, and drying area should be identified. Cigarette smokers in the home should be identified, cautioned against smoking in the presence of oxygen, and told of the increased health risks for the patient from second-hand smoke.

The evaluation of the physical environment cannot be underrated. Frequently, the RCP learns during the initial visit (and sometimes after the equipment has already been placed) that the home has problems that could affect the safety of the patient or the safe operation of the equipment. Some patients do not have electricity or they live in remote areas that experience frequent or prolonged power outages. Some homes have an accumulation of things the RCP considers to be rubbish but the owners consider to be valuable. Sometimes this accumulation takes up much of the free space in a home, blocking exits or walkways or posing a fire hazard. Some patients are unable to clean or maintain their homes because of illness or disability. Some have pets that are not housebroken but are allowed to move freely about the home. The home care RCP must use the skills of observation and persuasion to carefully determine which changes are necessary and which ones can be overlooked.

The Physical Assessment

The initial home visit may also include physical assessment of the patient. This assessment may be limited to pulse rate or breath sounds, for example, when a patient is receiving a one-time visit for a compressor-nebulizer setup, or it may be comprehensive, including oximetry, peak flow measurements, vital signs, auscultation, and other parameters.

The decision to perform a physical assessment (and the determination of its extent) usually depends on the patient's medical condition, the severity of this condition, the type of equipment that has been prescribed, and the preferences of the prescribing physician. For example, patients on home mechanical ventilation always require a detailed physical assessment, but home oxygen patients may not. Categorizing patients in this manner, however, is not always appropriate. Physical assessments should be performed on *any* patient the RCP deems necessary, regardless of the type of equipment being used, so long as the prescribing physician concurs. Conversely, a physical assessment should not be made simply because of the equipment a patient is going to use. The RCP must use decision-making skills in these cases and communicate his or her thoughts to the physician.

Table 2–7 outlines the parameters that are routinely evaluated during the initial physical assessment. Oxygen saturation by pulse oximetry may also be measured but only on the order of the patient's physician, because an oximeter is a prescription device. Some patients may also require capnography or basic pulmonary function testing; although they are not performed routinely, these tests are being used increasingly in home care. Whatever parameters are measured, the initial physical assessment is essential for establishing a baseline for the patient from which stasis, improvement, or decline can be measured.[12]

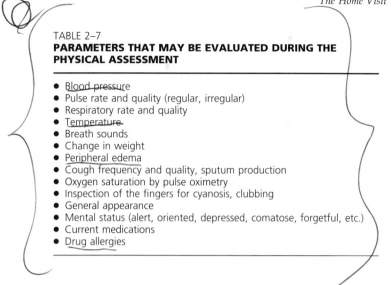

TABLE 2–7
PARAMETERS THAT MAY BE EVALUATED DURING THE PHYSICAL ASSESSMENT

- Blood pressure
- Pulse rate and quality (regular, irregular)
- Respiratory rate and quality
- Temperature
- Breath sounds
- Change in weight
- Peripheral edema
- Cough frequency and quality, sputum production
- Oxygen saturation by pulse oximetry
- Inspection of the fingers for cyanosis, clubbing
- General appearance
- Mental status (alert, oriented, depressed, comatose, forgetful, etc.)
- Current medications
- Drug allergies

Education and Training

Patient education and training is the primary duty of the home care RCP.[13] Most home care RCPs are employed by HME/RT providers, and a large part of the education and training they provide to the patient focuses on the safe and effective use of medical equipment. Whenever possible, patients should be encouraged and trained to manage the equipment themselves.

The patient and caregivers must be instructed not only in turning the equipment on and off, but also in cleaning, disinfecting, and maintaining it. They must understand the physician's intent for treatment; for example, the home oxygen therapy patient must understand the meaning of "continuous" use as opposed to "with exertion." Patients may also need education about the meaning of the ambiguous term "use as needed," as some home oxygen or nebulizer patients may not *know* when they need it. Sometimes patients may not know why the equipment has been prescribed for them, and the home care RCP will have to educate the patient about the indications as well as the contraindications for the prescribed therapy.

Patients and caregivers will need thorough instruction in troubleshooting equipment problems and steps to take in a power failure or emergency. They must also understand all safety issues related to the use of the equipment. Telephone numbers, instructions on reaching appropriate personnel after hours, and complaint procedures must also be provided.

The home care RCP will teach the patient and caregivers about more than equipment use. Symptom management, medication use and compliance, and even the pathophysiology of the patient's disease are important elements of the patient's education and training. During the initial visit, the home care RCP reviews the patient's use of cardiopulmonary medications, especially bronchodilators. This review might include proper measurement of the med-

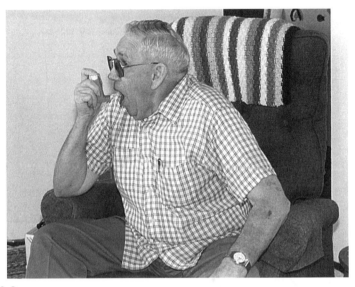

FIGURE 2–3
Proper method of using a metered-dose inhaler (MDI). The inhaler should be held in front of the open mouth or between the teeth with the mouth open. The patient should actuate the MDI and inhale slowly. Once the patient inhales as deeply as possible, he or she should then close the mouth and hold the breath for 10 sec (or as long as possible, if less than 10 sec). The patient should then exhale slowly.

ication, side effects, expected response to treatment, and proper storage of medications. Any allergies to medications should be identified.

The RCP often instructs a home care patient in using a compressor-nebulizer for aerosolized bronchodilators. The RCP also teaches patients to plan their nebulizer treatment times and helps set up a schedule if necessary. For example, a patient who has orders for compressor-nebulizer treatments four times a day may be scheduled to take them before breakfast, before lunch, before dinner, and again at bedtime. The home care RCP will not usually provide a metered-dose inhaler (MDI). These are more commonly provided by pharmacies or physicians' offices. The RCP may observe the patient using an MDI improperly during a home visit, however, and find it necessary to retrain the patient in the proper technique and prescribed dose. Figure 2–3 illustrates the recommended technique for using an MDI.

Patients should be questioned about any other medications they are taking, including dosages and frequencies. The patient should understand how to take the medications, and, if the RCP determines that the patient is confused about the medications, is not using them as prescribed, or is experiencing side effects, the physician should be notified. A visit to the pharmacist may also be recommended for a medication consultation. A visit by a home health nurse may also be helpful to the patient. Medication

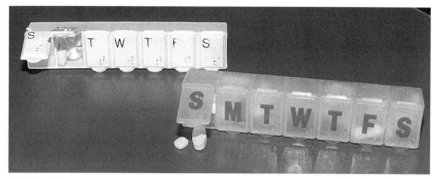

FIGURE 2–4
Medication scheduling device.

scheduling devices are very useful for helping patients take their medications at the proper times and on the proper days (Fig. 2–4).

The patient's education and training should also include symptom recognition related to the patient's pulmonary disease. Dyspnea, wheezing, chest pain, fatigue, and change in mucus production and consistency are signs and symptoms patients often overlook or are unable to control. Teaching patients to recognize the signs and symptoms that they experience in different situations will enhance their ability to either control them, treat them, or seek medical attention for them. Table 2–8 reviews common signs and symptoms experienced by home care patients and recommendations for self-management.

The RCP may also teach certain patients and caregivers to perform various respiratory care procedures like endotracheal suctioning or ventilator management. Table 2–9 lists respiratory care procedures commonly taught to home care patients. When teaching a patient these techniques, the home care RCP must be mindful of the differences in methods of technique performance at home as opposed to in the hospital. For example, a "clean technique" rather than a sterile technique is commonly used for oropharyngeal and endotracheal suctioning, and a suction catheter may be used repeatedly up to several days rather than once before discarding. Appendix 1 reviews common respiratory care procedures as they are taught in the home care setting.

Methods and Tools

The home care RCP has a dual challenge: trying to teach a lay person to use technical equipment and performing many of the functions of a credentialed health care professional. The education level of these caregivers can vary greatly, as does the level of willingness to provide care. Some may be squeamish at the thought of performing such procedures as suctioning

TABLE 2–8
**SIGNS AND SYMPTOMS AND MANAGEMENT STRATEGIES
TO REVIEW WITH THE HOME CARE PATIENT**

Sign, Symptom	Possible Cause	Management Strategy
Increased dyspnea	Equipment malfunction, patient not following MD's prescription, possible upper respiratory infection, anxiety, temperature	Check oxygen equipment, nebulizers; use O_2 or nebulizer as prescribed; implement breathing and energy conservation techniques; assessment by home care RCP; contact physician
Unexpected weight loss	Poor nutrition, increased dyspnea during eating, patient unable to prepare meals, improper use of diuretics	Contact physician, get assistance with meal preparation, use meals-on-wheels service, wear oxygen during meals, request evaluation with dietitian
Unexpected weight gain	Poor nutrition, use of oral steroids, improper use of diuretics, improper use of oxygen, possible congestive heart failure	Contact physician; review use of oral steroids, diuretics; review MD's prescription for oxygen; review food choices, salt intake; request evaluation with dietitian
Increased sputum production or change in sputum color	Possible upper respiratory infection, allergic response	Review cleaning and disinfection procedures, clean and disinfect equipment, take temperature, request RCP assessment, contact physician
Increased wheezing	Improper use of MDI, improper use of compressor-nebulizer, possible upper respiratory infection, allergic response	Review use of MDI and MD's prescription, review use of compressor-nebulizer and MD's prescription, request RCP assessment, contact physician
Change in sensorium	Not using oxygen as prescribed, using too much oxygen, improper medication use	Review MD's prescription for oxygen and medications, contact physician, call 911

or stoma care. They are expected to learn these procedures in very little time and then perform them without help from anyone. Fortunately, most patients and caregivers are able to learn and perform the required skills. It is common to see a tracheostomy patient whose family is able to perform tracheostomy tube changes deftly and safely while keeping a sterile field. Patients and their caregivers are taught to manage ventilator care, enteral feeding by food pump, and even IV care, sometimes all at the same time. Thorough education, training, and support are the keys to this type of success.

Everyone learns at a different speed and in a different way, and patience

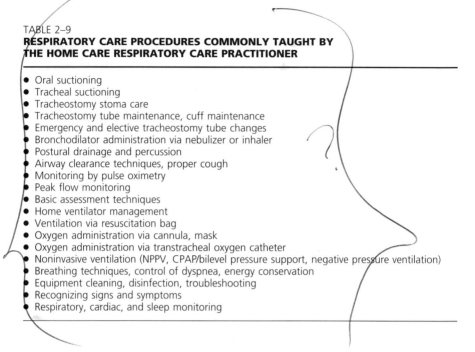

TABLE 2–9
RESPIRATORY CARE PROCEDURES COMMONLY TAUGHT BY THE HOME CARE RESPIRATORY CARE PRACTITIONER

- Oral suctioning
- Tracheal suctioning
- Tracheostomy stoma care
- Tracheostomy tube maintenance, cuff maintenance
- Emergency and elective tracheostomy tube changes
- Bronchodilator administration via nebulizer or inhaler
- Postural drainage and percussion
- Airway clearance techniques, proper cough
- Monitoring by pulse oximetry
- Peak flow monitoring
- Basic assessment techniques
- Home ventilator management
- Ventilation via resuscitation bag
- Oxygen administration via cannula, mask
- Oxygen administration via transtracheal oxygen catheter
- Noninvasive ventilation (NPPV, CPAP/bilevel pressure support, negative pressure ventilation)
- Breathing techniques, control of dyspnea, energy conservation
- Equipment cleaning, disinfection, troubleshooting
- Recognizing signs and symptoms
- Respiratory, cardiac, and sleep monitoring

on the part of the home care RCP is essential. Table 2–10 highlights various teaching tips that a home care RCP may find useful when training a patient or caregiver. The goal of the teaching process is to establish patient and caregiver competence in using the equipment, performing the required procedures, and managing the patient's medical condition, including calling for assistance when necessary. Patients should be involved in the education and training process whenever possible, even if they cannot perform the procedures themselves.[2,14-16]

TABLE 2–10
TEACHING TIPS FOR THE HOME CARE RESPIRATORY CARE PRACTITIONER

- Present only the necessary information
- Use only one instructor
- Limit the training sessions to 30 min, if possible
- Keep outside stimuli to a minimum (turn off television, radio; put the dog out, etc.)
- Limit the number of people at the training session to the patient and one or two family members or caregivers
- Present the information in the simplest terms possible; avoid medical jargon
- Use demonstration equipment
- Demonstrate the procedures *exactly* as they should be performed
- Repeat the demonstration as many times as necessary
- Ask the learner to perform a return demonstration
- Ask the learner to repeat the return demonstration until competency is established
- Leave written instructions and encourage the patient to review them
- Encourage the patient or caregivers to call with any questions or problems

Instructional materials are essential to the training process. Videotapes, booklets or manuals, and demonstration equipment are ideal tools. Patients' instructional materials should always be written in a style that is directed toward a lay person and not a clinician. Non–English speaking individuals should be provided with educational materials that either are written in a language they understand or are translated. User guides or other printed materials should be left at the patient's home whenever equipment is set up, giving the patient a reference if questions arise. All printed materials should include the name and 24-hour telephone number of the medical equipment provider.

The Plan of Service and the Respiratory Care Plan

The initial home visit finds the home care RCP performing many duties, including assessment of the patient (including psychosocial status), the home environment, and the presence and qualifications of family members or caregivers. The home care RCP sets up the prescribed equipment, instructs the patient and family members or caregivers in safe and effective use as well as routine care and maintenance and in summoning assistance if malfunction or breakdown occurs. At times, the home care RCP may also teach patients and others to perform certain respiratory care procedures. It is during the initial home visit that the home care RCP takes all collected information and formulates an individualized plan of service for equipment management. In certain cases, the home care RCP may also formulate a more detailed, clinically oriented respiratory care plan. These plans provide the framework under which certain activities are to be carried out during subsequent home visits so that the patient's chronic medical condition can be stabilized and a collaborative self-care regimen developed and implemented. The intensity of resources provided under a straightforward plan of service is measurably less than with a more complex respiratory care plan. The determination as to which patients are to receive the more intensive respiratory care plan is typically formalized in each company's mission and scope of service statement.

For example, a plan of service for equipment management may be totally appropriate for a patient referred for respiratory equipment who presents in a relatively stable state and appears quite capable of using the provided equipment in the prescribed manner. In this scenario, the HME/RT company may need to provide only those services needed to promote optimum and sustained equipment use. Initial education and training efforts focus on equipment use and operation, safety, infection control, trouble-shooting, and routine/preventive maintenance. The primary objective is to transfer responsibility to the patient for continued adherence to taught regimens. Subsequent home visits would be made to perform recommended quality control procedures on the respiratory equipment and to resupply exhausted inventories.

On the other hand, a more detailed respiratory care plan is appropriate for patients admitted to service who, unlike the previous hypothetical patient, present with a very fragile and unstable health status and express serious uncertainty about their ability to provide self-care. Such patients are at high risk for further deterioration and subsequent rehospitalization. Much the same can be said for patients who are already using high-tech respiratory equipment such as a mechanical ventilator or apnea monitor in a hospital, for whom discharge to home is being contemplated. In either of these scenarios, the appropriate approach is for the home care RCP to collaborate with the prescribing physician and, using data collected during the initial assessment, to formulate an intensive, individualized, clinically oriented respiratory care plan. The focus of the care plan is for the home care RCP to perform those activities necessary to bring the patient (or caregiver) to a higher level of self-sufficiency, forestall relapses, and promote clinical stability.[17] As part of the respiratory care plan, the home care RCP may measure and monitor vital signs and other symptoms, perform auscultation, measure blood oxygen saturations, conduct simple spirometry, perform chest physiotherapy, titrate equipment settings, teach cardiopulmonary resuscitation (CPR), and possibly even perform tracheal suctioning or tracheostomy tube changes. In addition to these "clinical goals," it will similarly be necessary for the home care RCP to carry out those activities designed to achieve equipment management goals, as mentioned in the discussion regarding a plan of service.

Aside from the fact that a respiratory care plan, unlike a plan of service, requires the signature of the prescribing physician, the main difference between a plan of service and a respiratory care plan is one of resource intensity. Simply stated, patients receiving home visits under a respiratory care plan require more time, effort, coordination, practitioner competency, and follow-up. By the same token, patients receiving home visits under a plan of service require much less time and effort, because the patient has assumed a much greater role in the management of his or her chronic medical condition. In either case, however, the plan that is ultimately formulated must be based upon clear and identifiable needs or problems. The activities, service, or care that is to be provided during home visits must be appropriate for addressing and resolving the identified needs or problems. Service or care plans must be periodically reviewed, updated, and, when necessary, revised. All material changes or revisions to respiratory care plans must be approved, in writing, by the prescribing physician. Figure 2–5 illustrates a respiratory care plan.

It is not uncommon for a patient who has received several home visits under a respiratory care plan to make significant improvements in his or her condition and ability to provide self-care. In this case, the home care RCP would make a determination that high-intensity home visits are no

RESPIRATORY CARE PLAN

PATIENT _____   PHYSICIAN_____

ADDRESS_____   ADDRESS_____

_____   _____

PHONE _____   _____
DATE_____

EQUIPMENT_____
PRESCRIPTION_____

HISTORY AND PHYSICAL

Primary dx:_____   Other dx:_____
Surgeries:_____   Family health hx:_____
Current medications:_____
Current symptoms:_____
Alcohol, drug use which affect cognition:_____
Ability to perform self-care, ADLs:_____
Physical limitations (ambulation, endurance, dyspnea on exertion, vision, hearing
etc):_____
Nutritional Status / Dietary Limitations:_____
Assessment of other care givers:_____
Other agencies involved in patient's care:_____

BP_____ HR_____ RR_____ Ht_____ Wt_____
O_2 sat (state activity, supplemental O_2) _____
Breath sounds_____
Cough, sputum production_____

PHYSICAL ENVIRONMENT

Safety of home for equipment and patient care (cleanliness, hazards,
barriers):_____
Grounded outlets, adequate electricity:_____
Adequate cleaning, storage facilities:_____
Telephone available:_____ Emergency exit plan:_____
Modifications needed:_____

Plan of Care /
Service:_____
_____
_____

Therapist:_____

Physician Signature / Date:_____

FIGURE 2–5
Sample respiratory care plan.

longer needed and would discharge the patient from clinical services. The patient would continue to receive home visits under a plan of service to ensure continued and optimum equipment management. In some companies, such home visits are made by specially trained equipment specialists rather than by a home care RCP.

Follow-Up Care

One of the services provided under both an equipment plan of service and the respiratory care plan is follow-up visits. These visits are made by the home care RCP or others to monitor the patient's progress toward defined goals and compliance with the service or care plan. Essential components of the follow-up visit are the physical and environmental assessments, quality control services on equipment, observation of patient and caregiver skills, and reeducation.

Visit Frequency

The frequency of follow-up visits is primarily determined by the needs of the patient, although some home care providers may have guidelines for visit frequencies based on the type of medical equipment the patient is using. Clinical practice guidelines and other published standards may recommend follow-up frequencies, particularly for equipment like mechanical ventilators.[15] A patient with complex medical or equipment needs may require a follow-up visit as frequently as daily for perhaps the first week. As the patient becomes more stable and adjusts to using the medical equipment, the home care RCP will be able to reduce the frequency of visits. For example, such a patient might be seen daily for the first week, twice a week for the next 2 weeks, and then weekly for the following 2 weeks. Eventually the visit frequency may be monthly, or even quarterly or less frequently, depending on the needs of the patient. The patient should be seen only as often as necessary and no less often than is clinically determined to be necessary. All home visits should be planned, coordinated, and meaningful.

Physical Assessment

During the follow-up visit the RCP may perform a physical assessment. This assessment includes taking vital signs and performing chest auscultation and possibly oximetry. Not every home care patient will need physical assessment; again, this is determined by the patient's needs. Some patients are very stable and others are being followed by home visiting nurses already performing such assessments. The home care RCP must evaluate each patient and decide whether care will be enhanced by such clinical services as physical assessment. For example, a patient who is discharged from the hospital with pneumonia and requires home oxygen therapy might benefit from physical assessment by the home care RCP. The patient could be monitored for change in heart rate with exertion and/or desaturation by pulse oximetry during that exertion. Chest auscultation and observation of sputum production can help evaluate the resolution of the pneumonia. The RCP's assessment during the follow-up visit can assist the physician in determining the patient's continuing need for oxygen therapy. It is important to remember, however, that any ongoing physical assessment the home care RCP feels is indicated, including oximetry, must be under the order of the patient's physician and embodied in a formal respiratory care plan.

Quality Control Services

The home care RCP will also provide quality control services on home medical equipment. Many types of home medical equipment have hour meters and contents gauges that are helpful in determining patient compliance. If a patient states that he is using the oxygen concentrator 24 hours per day, the RCP can check the hour meter to determine if this is indeed the case. The contents gauge on an oxygen tank can also help determine whether the patient is using the oxygen as much as prescribed.

Aside from evaluating patient compliance, HME/RT quality control services should include checking the home respiratory therapy equipment for proper function and performing any routine maintenance required by the equipment's manufacturer. For example, oxygen equipment should be checked for liter flow accuracy using a "liter meter" and for oxygen concentration using an oxygen analyzer. The home ventilator should have its settings and hour meter checked, filters changed, and battery charge evaluated. If the patient is responsible for any routine maintenance or cleaning, the equipment should be checked to verify that it is taking place. If equipment maintenance or cleaning is not being performed as originally instructed, the home care RCP should reinstruct as necessary.

Respiratory care procedures such as nebulizer treatments, suctioning, tracheostomy care, and the like should be observed for proper technique. If the procedures are not being performed satisfactorily, the home care RCP should review them with the patient and caregivers. Supplies should be evaluated for usage; improper usage may indicate an emergent problem, such as occurs when a patient uses more suction catheters than expected. This could indicate improper technique or an increased volume of secretions associated with respiratory infection. The home care RCP will assess the patient and contact the physician or retrain the patient or caregivers as indicated.

Revising the Plan of Service or the Respiratory Care Plan

The RCP should also evaluate whether the patient has met the goals previously set in a plan of service or respiratory care plan. For example, if one of the service goals for an oxygen patient is to have a functioning smoke detector in the home, the home care RCP will check for this. If the patient has been unable to meet this goal, the home care RCP must determine which service to provide to assist the patient. A patient whose goal is to properly fill his or her portable oxygen tank and use a higher flow rate when going out to the mailbox may demonstrate the ability to successfully fill the portable tank and adjust the tank's liter flow. If the patient goes out to the mailbox without oxygen because he or she feels uncomfortable filling the portable tank, the home care RCP can review the physician's prescription for oxygen therapy and the physical problems associated with hypoxemia. The home care RCP should review filling the portable tank and have the patient practice this procedure until the patient is confident of the ability to perform this task.

At the conclusion of the follow-up visit, the home care RCP determines which goals have been met, documents any new problems or needs, and works with the patient to establish new goals. The patient and the RCP then decide on a time for the next follow-up visit and the patient's tasks before that visit. The patient should be reminded of how to access the HME/RT company and encouraged to call the RCP with any questions, problems, or complaints.

Telephone Follow-Up

Another type of follow-up the home care RCP commonly performs is by telephone. A telephone follow-up is useful for monitoring patients who are stable and who show no compliance problems. It is also an acceptable way to monitor patients who decline home visits. Some patients do not wish to have anyone in their home, or they have so many other professionals making home visits that they do not want any more. Other patients may be too busy to see the home care RCP. The patient's right to decline home visits must be respected, and the home care RCP can try to monitor such patients by telephone.

During the telephone follow-up, the home care RCP can assess the patient by asking many of the same questions that are asked during a home visit. The patient can be asked about any changes in medical status or symptoms being experienced. The home care RCP should inquire about the patient's use of the equipment in relation to the physician's orders. For example, if the physician has ordered oxygen for continuous use, the home care RCP should ask the patient to estimate the amount of time the oxygen is being used. If the patient does not acknowledge that the oxygen is being used all the time, this should lead the RCP to ask additional questions to determine the patient's reasons for not following the prescription.

A telephone follow-up checklist can help prompt the home care RCP to ask the necessary questions and keep the telephone call on track. It can be easy to lose control of the conversation, with the patient discussing any number of unrelated subjects. Conversely, other patients are reluctant to volunteer information, and a checklist is useful in eliciting specific responses. Figure 2–6 is an example of a telephone follow-up checklist.

Discharging the Patient

Some patients require the services of a home care RCP for as long as they need home respiratory therapy equipment. For example, the ventilator-assisted patient requires a home care RCP on a long-term basis. Other patients do not require clinical respiratory services on an infinite basis. The home care RCP must decide who receives clinical respiratory services. Only those patients needing to be followed should be followed. Patients who no longer

---

TELEPHONE FOLLOW-UP CHECKLIST

PATIENT NAME_____   DATE_____

EQUIPMENT_____

How have you been feeling?_____
Are you having any new or unusual problems / symptoms?_____
If so, what are they?_____
Have you notified your physician of these symptoms?_____
If so, are you being treated for them?_____ How?_____

How often / much are you using your equipment?_____
Has your physician changed your liter flow / frequency?_____
If so, what is your new liter flow / frequency?_____
Which physician made this change?_____
Do you feel better when using your equipment?_____
Are you having any problems with the equipment?_____
How often are your cleaning or changing your nebulizer / humidifier / mask /
tubing?_____
How do you clean it?_____
How often do you disinfect your nebulizer / humidifier / mask /
tubing?_____
What solution do you use to disinfect your equipment?_____
How often do you discard this solution?_____

Do you need any additional equipment?_____
Do you need any supplies?_____

Do you have any questions about your equipment?_____
Do you have any comments or complaints about the service you are
*   receiving?_____*
_____
Services needed:_____
Follow-up plan:_____

Therapist:_____

FIGURE 2–6
Sample telephone follow-up checklist.

present a clinical need for follow-up should be discharged from these services.

Discharging a patient from clinical respiratory services is based on
certain criteria: (1) The patient dies, (2) the patient refuses the services, (3)
the patient is transferred to another HME/RT provider or health care facility,
or (4) the patient has achieved all realistic goals. The patient has the right
to refuse home visits, and in such an event there is no reason for the home
care RCP to follow him or her. However, the physician should be informed
whenever a patient refuses home visits.

The patient who has achieved the goals of the respiratory care plan
may be discharged because the medical need can no longer be justified by
the physician. Here the home care RCP performs a critical function. The
patient receives therapy only as long as is medically necessary, and the
home care RCP, through ongoing evaluation, can assist the physician in

determining the medical need. This is a benefit not only to the patient but to case managers and utilization review practitioners as well.

Consider the patient who is discharged from the hospital following treatment for pneumonia and for whom home oxygen therapy is ordered. The home care RCP evaluates the patient, establishes goals for the patient, and performs follow-up visits. One of the goals of therapy is to maintain an acceptable oxygen saturation at rest and with exertion.

The home care RCP monitors the patient's progress toward this goal. As progress is made, the physician may request that oximetry be performed on lowering amounts of oxygen, with the goal of maintaining an acceptable saturation on those lower amounts of oxygen. The home care RCP continues the home visits to monitor the patient's progress. It is to be hoped that the patient is recovering from the pneumonia and is requiring less oxygen. Once the goal of normal oxygen saturation on room air is reached, the physician will discontinue the oxygen therapy, and the patient will be discharged from clinical respiratory services. The home care RCP has played an essential role in justifying the treatment as well as in justifying that the treatment is no longer needed.

SUMMARY

The focus of health care is shifting away from acute care to that which is provided in the most cost-effective place of service, the home. Although home visits by an RCP are not currently reimbursed by Medicare, other payers see the value of RCPs in home care and *do* reimburse for their visits. These payers see that the home care RCP plays an important role in keeping the patient out of the hospital.

The home visit is a significant part of the home care RCP's job. The home visit is not a singular entity; rather, it is a complex series of events that, when taken as a whole, provide the RCP with a comprehensive view of the patient. This total picture is important because the home care RCP is responsible for developing and implementing a comprehensive respiratory care plan for the patient, not simply for delivering a piece of equipment.

The home care RCP is ideally positioned to monitor a patient's progress and identify emergent problems. In fact, the home care RCP is often the only professional following a patient at home. Patients look to the home care RCP for guidance and support. This is the essence of respiratory home care: providing patients with the training, support, and follow-up needed to understand their medical needs and to move toward independence and medical self-management.

> The home care RCP should visit patients when the patients need it for only as long as they need it and should continually update the respiratory care plan for as long as those visits are necessary.

REFERENCES

1. Home Care Advisory Panel: Guidelines for the Medical Management of the Home Care Patient. American Medical Association, Chicago, 1992, p 4.
2. Home Care Focus Group: AARC clinical practice guideline: Discharge planning for the respiratory care patient. Respiratory Care 40:1308, 1995.
3. Naylor, M et al: Comprehensive discharge planning for the hospitalized elderly. Ann Intern Med 12:999, 1994.
4. Make, BJ et al: Mechanical ventilation beyond the critical care unit: Report of a consensus conference of the American College of Chest Physicians. Chest Oct 1997, in press.
5. Thomas, VM et al: Caring for the person receiving ventilatory support at home: Care givers' needs and involvement. Heart Lung 21:180, 1992.
6. Smith, CE et al: Adaptation in families with a member requiring mechanical ventilation at home. Heart Lung 20:349, 1991.
7. Krider, SJ: Interviewing and respiratory history. In Wilkins, RL, Krider, SJ and Sheldon, RL (eds): Clinical Assessment in Respiratory Care, ed 3. Mosby-Year Book, St Louis, 1995, p 9.
8. American Thoracic Society: Standards of nursing care for adult patients with pulmonary dysfunction. American Review of Respiratory Diseases 1:231, 1991.
9. Fahr, LK: Psychosocial Consideration in the Care of the Adult with Chronic Pulmonary Disease. In Turner, J, McDonald, G and Larter, N (eds): Handbook of Adult and Pediatric Respiratory Home Care. Mosby-Year Book, St Louis, 1994, p 299.
10. Emery, CF: Psychosocial considerations among pulmonary patients. In Hodgkin, JE, Connors, GL and Bell, CW (eds): Pulmonary Rehabilitation: Guidelines to Success, ed 2. JB Lippincott, Philadelphia, 1993, p 279.
11. US Consumer Product Safety Commission: Safety for Older Consumers: Home Safety Checklist. US Government Printing Office, Washington, DC, 1986.
12. Wilkins, RL: Physical examination of the patient with cardiopulmonary disease. In Wilkins, RL, Krider, SJ and Sheldon, RL (eds): Clinical Assessment in Respiratory Care, ed 3. Mosby-Year Book, St Louis, 1995, p 47.
13. Dunne, PJ: The role of the RCP in home care. National Board for Respiratory Care (NBRC) Horizons 18:4, 1992.
14. Make, BJ: Collaborative self-management strategies for respiratory diseases in the home. Respiratory Care 39:566, 1994.
15. Turner, J: Patient compliance. In Turner, J, McDonald, G and Larter, N (eds): Handbook of Adult and Pediatric Respiratory Care, Mosby-Year Book, St Louis, 1994, p 357.
16. Home Care Focus Group: AARC clinical practice guideline: Long-term invasive mechanical ventilation in the home. Respiratory Care 401:1313, 1995.
17. McInturff, SL: A model plan of care. Home Health Care Dealer 35:43, 1993.

chapter 3

Home Care Equipment

Susan L. McInturff, RCP, RRT

Patrick J. Dunne, MEd, RRT

Teaching a patient to provide self-care using one or more items of respiratory therapy equipment is the major focus of the home care RCP. Patients are being discharged from the hospital much earlier during treatment of their disease, and they are often discharged needing medical equipment to help them continue that treatment once they are at home.

This chapter reviews the various types of respiratory and nonrespiratory home medical equipment (HME) the home care RCP may work with to assist patients in assuming responsibility for self-care at home. The chapter also includes discussion of the selection of the appropriate equipment to meet patients' needs, the delivery process, and the key elements of patient instruction.

The Home Medical and Respiratory Therapy Equipment Provider

Most home care RCPs providing home respiratory care are doing so as employees of a home medical and respiratory therapy equipment (HME/RT) provider. The HME/RT company provides a broad range of equipment and services, from simple ambulatory aids such as walkers, canes, and crutches to bathroom safety aids such as commodes and shower chairs to durable medical equipment (DME) such as hospital beds and wheelchairs. HME/RT companies also provide complex medical devices such as oxygen therapy equipment, home ventilators, IV pumps, and home sleep recorders. A majority of home care companies do not limit themselves to providing only home respiratory therapy equipment. Some companies do limit themselves to providing only DME such as beds, walkers, and wheelchairs, or they limit respiratory therapy equipment to oxygen and simple devices such as compressor-nebulizers.

HME/RT companies often categorize the types of equipment they provide by level of complexity:

1. **Category I:** No prescription needed; patient's life or health is not compromised by misuse of the equipment. May include all basic DME not legend-stamped by the US Food and Drug Administration.
2. **Category II:** Prescription needed; equipment is not considered life-supportive. Includes oxygen therapy equipment, nebulizers, suction machines, continuous positive airway pressure (CPAP) equipment, and oximeters.
3. **Category III:** Prescription needed; equipment is considered life-supportive. Includes apnea monitors, bilevel pressure support for respiratory failure, and invasive and noninvasive mechanical ventilators.

Depending on the level of complexity, an HME/RT company uses delivery technicians to set up most home care equipment. This may include home respiratory therapy devices such as oxygen equipment, compressor-nebulizers, and aspirators. Some companies train their delivery technicians to set up more complex equipment such as CPAP equipment or cardiorespiratory monitors. Using trained delivery technicians to set up most types of home respiratory therapy equipment is a cost-saving measure for the company because nonprofessional technicians are traditionally paid at a lower salary than are credentialed and licensed RCPs. However, in certain states, such a practice may be in conflict with respiratory therapy licensing statutes.

Home medical equipment is set up in one of two ways, depending on the type of equipment that has been ordered. Most commonly, the equipment is ordered by the referral source, and the delivery technician sets it up and teaches the patient to use it. If the delivery technician sets up respiratory therapy equipment, the home care RCP schedules an initial home visit. The initial visit is usually made within 24 to 48 hours of the setup, depending on the HME/RT company's policy. The home care RCP uses the initial home visit to assess the patient and ascertain whether the equipment meets the patient's needs. The home care RCP will also reinforce the instructions given to the patient during the setup and retrain as necessary.

If the respiratory therapy equipment being ordered is considered more technical and is classified in a higher category, the home care RCP is usually the one to deliver and set it up. The home care RCP will assess the patient, evaluate his or her needs, and develop a plan of treatment or service during this visit.

Home care RCPs should be familiar with all the categories of equipment the HME/RT company provides because they may be asked to set up equipment from any one of them. For example, the home care RCP may be asked to deliver and set up a wheelchair, walker, or other DME for a patient with whom they have a home visit scheduled. This eliminates the need of the HME/RT company to pay two employees to go to the patient's house, reducing the cost of delivery. The home care RCP can use this opportunity to evaluate the patient for his or her ability to use the equipment within the limitations of the pulmonary disease.

The home care RCP may also be called on to set up equipment not traditionally used in respiratory care. Breast pumps, continuous passive motion machines, or food pumps for enteral nutrition are examples of equipment home care RCPs might set up, provided they have the proper training. The home care RCP is often the only health care professional employed by a company. Most HME/RT companies do not employ both RCPs and nurses (although some companies have separate IV divisions that employ nurses to perform that function).

The Equipment Delivery

Once all the day's appointments have been scheduled, the home care RCP will select the equipment that will be needed from inventory. Some of this equipment will be brand new, such as a compressor-nebulizer or CPAP machine that is to be purchased by the patient. Some of the equipment will be drawn from the company's rental inventory. Regardless of whether the equipment is new or used, the home care RCP should always check the equipment for proper cleanliness and operation before loading it into his or her vehicle for delivery to the patient.

Patient-Ready Equipment

Ideally, the HME/RT company should have policies and procedures that govern making any piece of equipment "patient-ready." These policies and procedures outline the process for cleaning, disinfecting, and providing

TABLE 3–1
COMMONLY NEEDED EQUIPMENT AND SUPPLIES TO STOCK THE DELIVERY VEHICLE

Equipment	Supplies
Compressor-nebulizer	Medication nebulizers
CPAP machine, masks, and headgear	Filters for compressor-nebulizer
Pressure manometer for CPAP	Nasal cannulas, various types and sizes
Apnea monitor, electrode kit	Oxygen tubing, various lengths
Oxygen analyzer	Tubing connectors, various types
Liter meter	Nipple adapters
Respirometer	Concentrator filters, CPAP filters
Oximeter	
Blood pressure cuff	Adult and pediatric aerosol masks
Stethoscope	Miscellaneous adapters (15, 22 mm; oxygen bleed-in)
Small tools	Plastic bags, cleaning supplies

routine and preventive maintenance of the equipment. All equipment is checked to certify that it is functioning according to manufacturers' specifications, including power cords, fuses, and on/off switches. The equipment is logged into the company's equipment maintenance system to document that the appropriate level of service has been performed. New equipment is returned to its original carton and resealed, and rental equipment is usually bagged. The equipment is then placed in the company's designated patient-ready area.

The home care RCP might assume that all bagged and boxed equipment is ready for use. However, it is wise to double-check the equipment. New equipment simply may not work; in older equipment, a filter may not have been replaced, or the equipment may not have been thoroughly cleaned. It is certainly better to make this determination before giving such equipment to a patient. A good rule of thumb for the home care RCP is to *always check the equipment before leaving the company premises.*

Stocking the Delivery Vehicle

The home care RCP should carry commonly used equipment and supplies in the delivery vehicle. Keeping extra equipment and supplies on hand is useful because the home care RCP may be called for a setup while he or she is out in the field. Being ready eliminates the need to return to the office to pick up the necessary equipment. Any patient-ready equipment kept in the home care RCP's vehicle should be separated from equipment that has been picked up from a patient, has not been cleaned, or is in some other way not ready for patient use. This is most easily accomplished by keeping patient-ready equipment in clear plastic bags. Table 3–1 lists commonly needed equipment and supplies that the home care RCP should keep stocked in his or her delivery vehicle. Disposable supplies such as cannulas and tubing should remain unopened in the original packaging to identify them as unused.

The home care RCP should carry tools and supplies needed to service and adjust equipment such as oxygen analyzers, liter meters, and screwdrivers (Phillips and flathead types and extra-small for CPAP pressure adjustments). It is also very useful to carry cleaning supplies in the event that a piece of equipment must be used on another patient. The home care RCP should have some means of recording on-the-road equipment cleaning and servicing. Equipment that has been cleaned should be placed in plastic bags to differentiate it from dirty equipment.

The home care RCP's delivery vehicle must also be stocked with an Infection Control Kit. This kit should include nonsterile gloves, face masks, protective eyewear, gowns, and special bags (generally red) in which to put these items after use to designate them as hazardous waste. A no-rinse disinfectant hand cleaner is an essential staple and should be kept in a convenient location for use when the home care RCP is unable to wash his or her hands at a patient's home. Refer to Chapter 5 of this book for a more complete review of infection control.

Extra paper supplies should be carried in the delivery vehicle. Such supplies include extra sets of patient instructional materials, charting forms, and delivery invoices. Stickers or business cards with the HME/RT company's telephone number should also be carried. Extra writing materials come in handy for taking notes when the home care RCP is paged on the road.

The home care RCP's delivery vehicle should also carry standard vehicle safety supplies such as a tire jack, spare tire, road flares, snow chains (where applicable), and a flashlight. A full set of maps or map books covering the home care RCP's territory is essential. A cellular phone is useful for summoning assistance in the event of vehicular problems. Home care RCPs should carry their driver's license, their license or certificate to practice respiratory care (where applicable), automobile registration, and proof of automobile insurance at all times.

The Equipment

The home care RCP works with many types of respiratory therapy equipment to treat patients with chronic cardiopulmonary diseases. The home care RCP may also set up home medical equipment not traditionally used in respiratory care, such as walking aids, bathroom safety aids, enteral food pumps, and phototherapy lights. This section reviews the most common types of medical equipment provided by home care RCPs.

Home Oxygen Therapy Equipment

Oxygen therapy equipment is probably the most frequently ordered home respiratory therapy equipment. It is no wonder, when chronic obstructive pulmonary disease (COPD) has been identified as the second leading cause of long-term disability and is ranked as the fifth leading cause of death in the United States.[1] Three different types of equipment are used to deliver home oxygen therapy: the liquid oxygen system, oxygen concentrator system, and compressed gas systems. Each system has advantages and disadvantages, and the decision as to which system should be selected is based on the needs of the patient and the physician's order. The need for portability and for oxygen conservation plays a significant role in equipment selection.[2]

Oxygen systems are stationary, portable, or ambulatory. A *stationary* oxygen system is considered to be stationary because of its size and weight; it is placed in a particular location in the patient's home and left there as the patient's primary source of oxygen. A *portable* oxygen system is small but heavy enough to usually require its transportation in a wheeled cart. Small steel or aluminum compressed oxygen cylinders are typically used as portable systems. An *ambulatory* system is also small, but it is light enough for the patient to carry on his or her person, usually by a shoulder strap. Many home care professionals use the terms "portable" and "ambulatory" interchangeably when speaking about oxygen systems intended for use primarily when the patient is away from the stationary source.

Liquid Oxygen

Liquid oxygen systems use a special thermos-type tank known generically as a dewar to store the oxygen in its liquid state at −273°F. The liquid oxygen flows up through a draw tube and travels through warming coils. This travel causes the liquid oxygen to evaporate; the resultant gas passes through a flow control valve and on to the patient. The flow control valve can deliver flows from ¼ to 15 liters per minute (L/min), depending on the valve. The liquid oxygen tank is periodically refilled by the HME/RT company, depending on the size of the tank and the patient's flow rate. A standard-size liquid oxygen (LOX) stationary tank would be refilled approximately once per week when the patient is using 2 L/min continuously.

The LOX system is an ideal choice for the patient requiring a stationary and ambulatory system. The LOX system includes a small, lightweight tank the patient can fill whenever the need arises. This portable tank is light enough for most patients to carry on their shoulder, and some patients carry it in a backpack. Patients who find the small tank too heavy to carry can put it in a wheeled cart. A standard-size ambulatory tank will give the patient about 15 hours of use when used at a flow rate of 1 L/min, 8 hours at a flow rate of 2 L/min. Figure 3–1 illustrates a LOX stationary and ambulatory system.

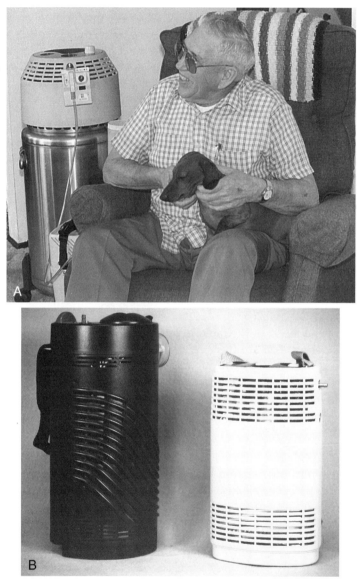

FIGURE 3–1
(*A*) Stationary liquid oxygen (LOX) reservoir. (*B*) Two types of ambulatory LOX units.

The primary advantage of the LOX system is that it allows patients to be away from their stationary tank for longer periods than do other systems. Another advantage is that patients can fill the small tanks as frequently as they wish. The LOX system is also very quiet and requires no electricity to power it. Most patients can learn to fill the small tank without difficulty, and the virtually unlimited access to ambulatory oxygen and longer use times may encourage patients to leave the home more frequently.

LOX systems have several disadvantages. Oxygen in its liquid state is extremely cold and requires special handling by the HME/RT company's delivery personnel. Gloves and protective eyewear are required when transfilling the stationary tank to protect the delivery technician from burns that occur when liquid oxygen contacts skin. The tanks themselves are more costly for the HME/RT company to own and operate compared with other oxygen delivery systems, and the company must also factor in the cost of having to make repeated deliveries to its oxygen clients.

Also, the LOX system is somewhat wasteful because of evaporative loss. The liquid oxygen in the tank is evaporating at a steady rate whether or not the tank is being used. Warmer room temperatures and frequent transfilling of the small tank causes even more evaporative loss. Some insurance companies (particularly Medicare) do not pay for the actual oxygen contents; they pay only for the rental of the tank. Evaporative loss of contents paired with the lack of reimbursement and the need to make repeated deliveries can make the provision of LOX systems less than attractive to some HME/RT companies.

Finally, some patients find that filling the small tank is too difficult. Others find the noise that occurs during the filling process too frightening or unbearable. Patients must be able to properly connect the small LOX tank to the stationary LOX tank, open a vent to start the filling process, observe both tanks during the fill, and stop the process before overfilling occurs. Patients must also be prepared to react if the couplers on either tank freeze open. Patients must be able to accurately read contents gauges on both tanks, and this is especially important when using the small tank. They must be able to determine how long their small tank will last when they are away from home to prevent running out of oxygen before they return.

The home care RCP must consider all of the advantages and disadvantages when selecting liquid oxygen for a patient. Sometimes it is the only choice, as is the case for the patient who has inadequate or no electricity. Patients who do not require ambulatory oxygen and who do not have an environmental limitation like electricity may not need liquid oxygen, but, rather, a less expensive method.

Oxygen Concentrator

An oxygen concentrator is an electrically powered machine that draws in room air, separates the nitrogen from it, and delivers the remaining oxygen

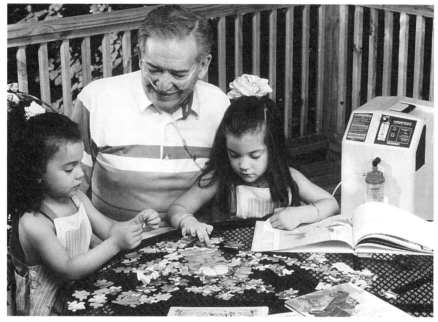

FIGURE 3–2
Oxygen concentrator. (Courtesy of Nellcor Puritan Bennett, Pleasanton, CA.)

to the patient. Oxygen concentrators are now capable of delivering flow rates as low as ¼ L/min up to 6 L/min. Oxygen concentrators are used in the home as the patient's primary, stationary source of oxygen. Figure 3–2 shows one type of oxygen concentrator used at home.

The primary advantage of oxygen concentrators is their ability to provide a continuous source of oxygen as long as electricity is available, eliminating the need for repeated deliveries for refills. The concentrator is easy to operate and requires little maintenance by the patient.

The oxygen concentrator has some disadvantages. It is rendered inoperable during an electrical power failure, requiring the placement of an alternate source of oxygen in the home (usually a compressed oxygen cylinder). Also, the concentrator's compressor makes noise that some patients find very disturbing. In addition, the concentrator generates heat during operation, which can increase the ambient temperature of the room; if a concentrator is placed in a small room with little ventilation, the patient may find the increased room temperature uncomfortable. An oxygen concentrator will increase a patient's utility bill (by an estimated $25 or more per month), a factor that should not be overlooked when the user has limited financial resources.

Oxygen concentrators require routine testing by the HME/RT company to ensure proper function. Most concentrators do not have an oxygen concentration indicator to alert the user of subnormal oxygen concentration or flow. Such problems can be hazardous to the patient. Newer concentrators come equipped with such indicators, and older concentrators can be retrofitted with these monitoring devices. In the absence of an oxygen concentration indicator, the HME/RT company must routinely analyze the concentration and test the flow rate for accuracy, a task that many home care RCPs perform during their home visits. Oxygen concentrators must also be periodically removed from service for more extensive maintenance.

An oxygen concentrator is an ideal choice as a stationary oxygen source for the patient who is home bound or who requires a stationary and *portable* system. An oxygen concentrator is very economical for the HME/RT provider, requiring only periodic service calls for preventive maintenance. Some companies place concentrators *and* LOX systems in a patient's home, the former as a stationary system and the latter for portability. This minimizes the number of deliveries the company must make to either refill the LOX system or replace empty cylinders.

Compressed Oxygen Systems

The hospital-based RCP is quite familiar with high-pressure compressed oxygen tanks. Such tanks are used in home oxygen therapy as well. Large H tanks (244 cubic feet) are used as stationary sources of oxygen, primarily as emergency backup systems to oxygen concentrators. An H tank is not commonly used as a primary stationary source of oxygen because of its limited contents; for example, a patient using oxygen continuously at 2 L/min would need an H tank replaced every 2 days, requiring very frequent deliveries or placement of several tanks in the home at the same time.

Small E- and D-sized compressed oxygen tanks are commonly used for portable systems. These tanks are made of either steel or lightweight aluminum and are usually moved on a wheeled cart. Aluminum D tanks can also be carried in a shoulder bag. Very small cylinders, M6, are also used but usually only with an oxygen conserving device. The small size of the M6 tank allows only a very limited use time, requiring the patient to carry more than one cylinder or allowing very short periods away from home. Figure 3–3 illustrates several portable compressed oxygen systems.

Using compressed oxygen tanks for portability does not allow patients as many hours of use as does the LOX ambulatory tank at the same flow rate. Because of this limitation, a compressed oxygen portable system may be most appropriate for the patient who does not require more than 3 to 4 hours of portable oxygen per week, such as the patient who leaves home only for doctor visits.

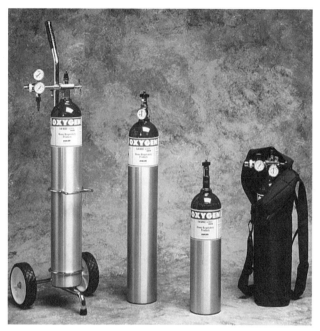

FIGURE 3–3
Different sizes of portable oxygen cylinders.

Oxygen Conserving Devices

One way to increase the use time of an oxygen tank, whether liquid or compressed gas, is to use an oxygen conserving device (OCD) with the tank. OCDs reduce the amount of oxygen used, making a portable or ambulatory tank last longer and greatly increasing the length of time between refill deliveries for a stationary tank.

The conventional continuous flow oxygen system is considered wasteful because oxygen is flowing even during a patient's exhalation phase, when it is not being used. OCDs provide oxygen on inspiration only and are capable of adequately oxygenating a patient at much lower flow rates.[3] Three types of OCDs are in use today: the reservoir cannula, the pulsed-dose system, and the transtracheal oxygen catheter.

Reservoir Cannula

The first OCD to be developed, which is also the least expensive, is the reservoir cannula. This device uses a small reservoir to store the continuously flowing oxygen during the patient's exhalation, making it available as a bolus during inspiration. (This concept is similar to that of the nonrebreathing mask.) The higher concentration of oxygen inhaled from the reservoir allows for a lower overall liter flow. Therein lies the conservation: The lower the flow rate, the longer the oxygen tank will last. Reservoir cannulas are reported to present an average oxygen savings of 66 percent.[3]

Two types of reservoir cannulas are in use: the "mustache" cannula and the pendant cannula. Despite their oxygen conserving capabilities, reservoir cannulas are not widely used because of their somewhat conspicuous appearance. These cannulas are also heavier than conventional nasal cannulas, making them uncomfortable to wear.[3] Some patients are willing to wear reservoir cannulas for limited periods when they are not in public.

Another disadvantage to using the reservoir cannula is that, although it is the least expensive OCD, it is quite a bit more expensive than a conventional cannula. Most insurance companies do not pay extra for cannulas and tubing, considering these items to be included in the monthly rental price of the oxygen system. Patients using reservoir cannulas may have to pay for them personally.

Any patient being considered for this or any other type of OCD should be evaluated by pulse oximetry to determine whether the lower flow rate is adequate. It is important to evaluate oxygen saturation during rest and especially during activity when using a reservoir cannula or other OCD.[3]

Pulsed-Dose Systems

A fairly recent advancement in oxygen conservation is the pulsed-dose demand system. This type of OCD is an electromechanical device that administers a "pulse" of oxygen, or, rather, a small bolus, at the beginning of a patient's inspiration. Having a small bolus of oxygen, approximately 35 mL, delivered only at the beginning of inspiration (as opposed to a continuous flow) results in a significant reduction in the amount of oxygen used. Pulsed-dose OCDs have been reported to reduce the amount of oxygen used by 50 to 75 percent.[3]

Pulsed-dose oxygen conserving devices typically use one of two competing technologies: rate-responsive devices that *do not* deliver oxygen on every breath or demand delivery systems that do. Either technology can be used with both compressed oxygen systems and liquid oxygen tanks (Fig. 3–4). Most pulsed-dose devices are equipped with a switching mechanism that will allow the patient to convert to a continuous flow if needed. Some pulsed-dose OCDs will switch to continuous flow if an inspiration is not detected within a specific length of time. It is also important that the home care RCP determine that the use of pulsed-dose conserving devices does not have an adverse effect on a particular patient's oxygen saturation levels.

OCDs may be powered by a rechargeable internal battery or may be replaceable, and patients using them must learn to maintain and recharge the battery. The patient must also know what to do if the battery loses its charge while in use. Some pulsed-dose units make an audible "clicking" noise when their demand valves open, which the user may find annoying or conspicuous. Most patients are willing to ignore this, especially when

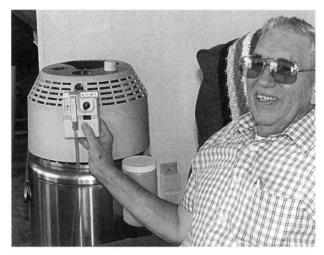

FIGURE 3–4
Pulsed-dose oxygen conserving device (OCD). OCDs can be used on both LOX and compressed oxygen tanks.

they learn that the tank will provide 10 to 20 hours or more of use. This use time is dependent on the size of the tank and the patient's respiratory rate.

The use of pulsed-dose conserving devices can greatly enhance a patient's mobility. They are not used as frequently as they could be, however, because many insurance companies, including Medicare, do not reimburse oxygen providers for the device. Some HME/RT companies find it financially difficult to provide a patient with a piece of equipment costing several hundred dollars with no reimbursement. Other companies see the financial savings in providing a piece of equipment that reduces the number of deliveries needed to refill a patient's oxygen tank. The home care RCP must be aware that some HME/RT companies will charge the patient for the rent or purchase of the OCD and take that into consideration when recommending such a device for a patient.

Transtracheal Oxygen Systems

The transtracheal oxygen system (TTOS) is an invasive method of oxygen conservation. Oxygen is delivered directly into the trachea via a small Silastic catheter that has been inserted percutaneously (Figs. 3–5A and 3–5B). Because oxygen is delivered directly into the trachea, the anatomical deadspace of the nasopharynx is bypassed. Oxygen may be flowing through the TTOS catheter continuously, but the overall flow rate needed to oxygenate the patient is reduced because part of the flow is not wasted in filling the deadspace of the nose and larynx. The reduction in required oxygen flows has been reported to be as much as 50 percent at rest and 30 percent with exercise.[3,4] Further oxygen savings occurs by pairing the TTOS system with a pulsed-dose oxygen conserving device.

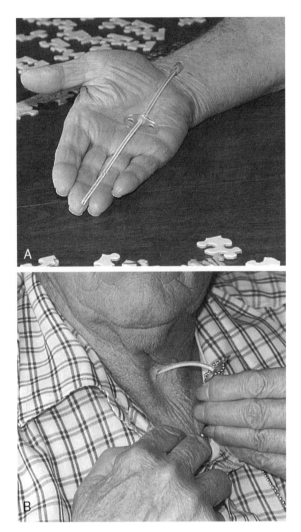

FIGURE 3–5
(*A*) Transtracheal oxygen catheter.
(*B*) Transtracheal oxygen catheter
inserted into the trachea.

Placement of the transtracheal catheter is a relatively simple procedure that is frequently undertaken in the physician's office. It requires only a local anesthetic and a very small incision. The patient must return to the physician's office for catheter changes for a few weeks, after which the stoma, or tract, will have matured enough for the patient to change the catheter himself or herself.

The TTOS offers several advantages over conventional oxygen administration via nasal cannula. The catheter is held securely in the neck by a chain, reducing accidental disruption in oxygen delivery such as occurs with a nasal cannula during sleep. Use of a TTOS eliminates the rubbing and irritation of the ears, face, and nares that occur with nasal cannula use, and patients are less likely to interrupt their oxygen flow to relieve such irritation. Many patients find the catheter to be a more cosmetically appealing alternative to the nasal cannula, particularly when it can be hidden beneath a shirt collar. This inconspicuousness can increase compliance in patients who will not wear a nasal cannula in public. Patients with refractory hypoxemia requiring increasingly higher flows of oxygen to maintain acceptable saturation levels can be successfully treated with lower flow rates via a TTOS.[3,5] Other reported benefits include an improved sense of smell and taste, improved sleep, and increased exercise tolerance.[3,4]

The TTOS has some disadvantages. An invasive procedure, even one as simple as the percutaneous insertion of the catheter, places the patient at risk for complications such as infection, bronchospasm, and subcutaneous emphysema.[3,5] The catheter requires daily maintenance, including instillation of saline into the catheter, insertion of a cleaning rod, and periodic removal and reinsertion of a new catheter. These procedures are required to prevent formation of mucus balls that can obstruct the catheter. Careful patient selection is necessary because not every patient who might benefit from the TTOS is a good candidate. Some patients are unwilling or unable to perform the cleaning and replacement procedures; the patient must be particularly motivated to care for the catheter as instructed.[3,5]

Conventional Oxygen Delivery Devices

Patients requiring home oxygen therapy use the same types of delivery devices seen in the hospital. A great majority of home oxygen patients use a nasal cannula with up to 50 feet of oxygen tubing attached to their stationary oxygen system. There should be enough tubing to allow the patient access to all the areas of his or her home that are used.

Occasionally the home care RCP will encounter a patient with a house that is very large or has more than one story, and 50 feet of tubing is not long enough. The obvious solution is to increase the length of the tubing. This is not recommended, however, because the added length of tubing increases the resistance in the tubing to oxygen flow. The increased resistance reduces the flow, and the patient will receive a *lower* flow rate than that set on the stationary system. For those patients for whom 50 feet of tubing is not enough, a second stationary system may be useful. Another alternative is for the patient to use a portable or ambulatory system to access those areas of the home not reached by the stationary system.

Oxygen masks are used for some home oxygen patients, but not very frequently. Generally, patients requiring the higher concentrations delivered by oxygen masks are too ill to remain at home. There are patients, however, who will require oxygen masks at home. Usually they are terminally ill, are not going to be hospitalized, and have refractory hypoxemia. These patients use high-flow oxygen as a comfort measure.

Should the home care RCP need to set up an oxygen mask on a patient at home, it will most often be a simple mask. A simple mask is more easily set up because it requires flow rates of 5 to 10 L/min, common flows found on most home oxygen equipment. Partial, nonrebreathing, and Venturi masks are more difficult to use because of the higher flow rates they require. It is much more difficult to provide oxygen equipment capable of delivering those high flows. Either the stationary tank will need to be refilled more frequently, more than one tank will need to be used, or larger tanks will be necessary.

Bubble humidifiers are also used on oxygen systems for a select group of patients. Studies have shown that humidifiers are not necessary for patients using less than 4 L/min.[6] However, patients complaining of a dry mouth, nasal irritation, or nosebleeds may benefit from having a humidifier in-line with their oxygen. The patient must be instructed to use distilled or boiled water when filling the humidifier, to routinely clean and disinfect the humidifier, and to troubleshoot for the leaks that are common with humidifier use.

Patient Instruction

The home care RCP will have to instruct or review the instructions the patient has received regarding the proper use of the oxygen therapy equipment. Some key elements should be covered during this training.

The Prescription.

A patient should not leave his or her pharmacy without understanding how to take the medications the doctor has prescribed. Similarly, a patient must understand how to use his or her oxygen as prescribed. The home care RCP must advise the patient of the physician's prescription, including the flow rate to use at rest, at night, and with activity; the number of hours per day to use the oxygen; and acceptable times to not use the oxygen.[7]

This task can be difficult if the physician's intent for treatment is unclear, such as when oxygen is ordered "prn." The physician may tell a patient to use the oxygen "when the patient thinks he or she needs it," but the patient may not know when that is. Some patients think they need to use the oxygen *after* performing an activity that causes them to become short of breath. Other patients will use the oxygen all the time, when they actually need it only during exercise. Still other patients, when given this option, may decide they *never* need it. The home care RCP may need to contact the patient's physician for clarification if it is unclear as to when or how much oxygen the patient should use.

Patients having oxygen prescribed for continuous use must understand

TABLE 3–2
COMMON TROUBLESHOOTING TECHNIQUES FOR HOME OXYGEN EQUIPMENT

- Set cannula into a glass of water and watch for bubbling.
- Check contents gauge on tank.
- Check flow setting on oxygen source.
- Check on/off switch if there is no flow.
- Check all tubings for kinks, connections.
- Check washable filter on concentrator for clogging.
- Check humidifier bottle for leaks at threads, cross-threading.
- Remove or replace humidifier.
- If concentrator spontaneously stops, check positioning of machine and make sure it has 18 inches of space on each side (concentrator can overheat without sufficient ventilation, causing it to quit running spontaneously).
- Check circuit breaker on back of concentrator; push back in if it has popped.
- Check power cord on concentrator to be sure it is plugged in.
- Check to be sure light switch is turned on if concentrator is plugged into outlet controlled by that light switch.

that "continuous" means just that. For some patients, however, the word continuous means they wear it until they shower, eat, or shop. The home care RCP should counsel patients about the physical effects of removing the oxygen when they need it the most, particularly during periods of exertion. Many patients are surprised to learn that they should keep the oxygen on when they get into the shower or that it can be harmful to run out to the mailbox without it.

In addition to those patients who do not wear their oxygen enough, the RCP will also encounter those patients who increase or decrease their oxygen flow rate above or below the amount the physician has prescribed. All home oxygen patients should be cautioned against changing their oxygen flow rate without first consulting their physician. The patient might be advised that changing the liter flow can be likened to taking more or less heart medication than prescribed: Both situations can have detrimental effects.

The Equipment

The home care RCP should always review the proper operation of the oxygen therapy, including how to turn the equipment on and off, how to read contents gauges, and how to estimate the length of time the portable or ambulatory tank will last. Patients must also be taught to perform any routine maintenance procedures for which they will be responsible, such as cleaning filters and disinfecting humidifiers. The home care RCP should review the method of filling the ambulatory LOX tank or changing regulators on empty compressed oxygen cylinders.

Patients should always be taught to perform any minor troubleshooting procedures applicable to the oxygen system being used, like what to do if they feel they are not getting oxygen flow or how to reset the circuit breaker on a concentrator. Table 3–2 reviews common troubleshooting techniques for home oxygen equipment. Printed instructions that include troubleshooting techniques and the HME/RT provider's 24-hour telephone number should always be left with the patient. Patients should be encouraged to call their oxygen provider at any time with questions, problems, or complaints.

Oxygen Safety

The home care RCP will also review the safe handling and storage of oxygen. Although oxygen is a hazardous material, it is safe when handled with care. Oxygen is not combustible but does support burning, so patients should be cautioned to stay away from sparks or open flames. Oxygen equipment must also be kept away from open flames, preferably in another room. Patients who smoke should be discouraged from doing so or advised to at least turn off the oxygen, remove the nasal cannula, and step outside if they insist on smoking. Of course, these patients should be reminded of the physical complications of interrupting their oxygen therapy. Other smokers should also be instructed to step outside to smoke. A "No Smoking—Oxygen in Use" sign should be posted on the front door of the home to alert visitors to the presence of oxygen equipment.

Any oxygen system in use must be secured to prevent its falling over. This is particularly important when compressed oxygen tanks are being used. An H tank should always be secured in a stand or "collar," and smaller cylinders should be secured in a cart or laid on the floor. Patients should be instructed to keep cylinder valves closed when tanks are not in use, to store tanks in a well-ventilated area, and to avoid exposing compressed oxygen tanks to extremes in temperature. Patients should also be advised to use caution when transporting oxygen tanks to avoid dropping or hitting cylinders. It is recommended that tanks not be placed in the trunk of a car but be transported inside the car. This precaution is because of the high temperatures that can build up in a car's trunk, the greater possibility of the presence of petroleum products like oil or gasoline, and the potential of the trunk's being an oxygen-enriched atmosphere should the oxygen tank leak.

The home care RCP should caution the patient against the use of petroleum- or alcohol-based products like petroleum jelly, hair oils, or aerosol sprays. For example, patients have been known to use petroleum jelly (mentholated) around their nares to reduce the irritation of nasal cannula prongs or to lubricate the threads on an oxygen tank to help seal leaks at the point of attachment of the humidifier. These commonly used products are combustible, however, and the oxygen supports combustion. Add a spark from a cigarette, an electric razor, a sparking toy, or other source, and the oxygen-enriched atmosphere around the patient can ignite very easily. Table 3–3 lists safety tips for home oxygen systems.

Oxygen equipment, when used properly and as prescribed, is a very important part of many home care patients' treatment. If the home care RCP

TABLE 3–3
HOME OXYGEN SAFETY TIPS

- Always keep cylinders in carts or tank collars.
- Small cylinders should be laid on the floor if not secured in a cart.
- Avoid knocking cylinders together (this can create sparks).
- Remove and avoid combustible materials (i.e., petroleum jelly, hair oil, hair and other aerosol sprays, petroleum-based skin lotions, grease).
- Remove and avoid sources of ignition (i.e., hair dryers, electric razors, open flames, heaters, sparking toys, lit cigarettes).
- Place oxygen source at least 6 feet away from flames or other sources of ignition.
- Do not place oxygen tanks in the trunk of the car.
- Keep oxygen tanks in a well-ventilated area to prevent the buildup of an oxygen-enriched atmosphere.
- Use "No Smoking—Oxygen in Use" signs to alert others to the presence of oxygen in the home.
- When filling a LOX portable tank, avoid contact with the stream of liquid oxygen that is seen at the vent when the tank is full.

does his or her part to properly evaluate, instruct, and conduct follow-up, the patient can have a safe and positive experience with oxygen.

Aerosol Therapy

Many of the patients with COPD and asthma treated in the home receive nebulized bronchodilator therapy. Other patients receive aerosolized pentamidine via a high-output compressor. Patients who have undergone tracheotomies and laryngectomies may need bland aerosol therapy. The home care RCP must be prepared to set up various types of aerosol delivery devices for patients with varying aerosol needs.

Compressor-Nebulizers

Most patients requiring bronchodilator therapy are taught to use a metered-dose inhaler (MDI), and many can use an MDI quite successfully. There are some patients for whom the MDI is not the delivery method of choice, however. For example, the pediatric patient may be too young to perform the breathing maneuvers required with MDI use. The COPD patient may be too dyspneic or incapable of taking a deep breath or may be unable to hold his breath as long as necessary for maximal particle deposition. Patients with arthritis in their hands or with reduced hand strength may be unable to actuate the MDI. Others are unable to use the MDI correctly no matter how many times they are instructed. All of these patients would benefit from using a compressor-nebulizer.

   The compressor-nebulizer is a small electric- or battery-powered oil-free device that provides a flow of compressed air to power a medication

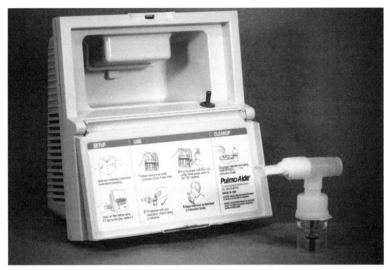

FIGURE 3–6
Compressor-nebulizer.

nebulizer (Fig. 3–6). Compressor-nebulizers used in home care are capable of putting out flow rates of 8 to 15 L/min at about 20 psi. These devices are easy for the user to operate and maintain. Many patients use a compressor-nebulizer to take their bronchodilator treatments while they are at home and MDIs when they are not.

Patient Instruction

The home care RCP setting up a compressor-nebulizer will teach the patient to assemble the medication nebulizer, to accurately measure and put medications into the nebulizer, and to take a treatment. The patient must learn to clean and disinfect the medication nebulizer (nebulizers are reused many times before needing replacement), replace compressor filters, and troubleshoot for minor problems (Table 3–4). The home care RCP will also review

TABLE 3–4
PATIENT TROUBLESHOOTING TIPS FOR COMPRESSOR-NEBULIZERS

- If the unit will not turn on, check the power cord.
- If the unit has been in a cold environment and will not turn on, rock the power switch on and off several times (this should free the compressor).
- Check the nipple adapter on the compressor to ensure it has no leaks.
- Check the medication nebulizer to be sure it has been assembled properly.
- Check the tiny jet holes to be sure they are not clogged.
- Inspect the compressor's filter; change it if it looks gray.
- Replace the medication nebulizer.

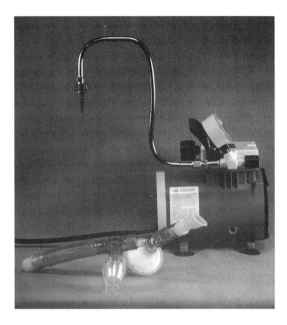

FIGURE 3–7
Tabletop compressor.

treatment schedules based on the physician's order, proper response to treatment, and common side effects of the medication. For patients also using an MDI, the home care RCP may observe their techniques and retrain as indicated.

High-Output Compressors

The high-output compressor, sometimes called a "tabletop" compressor, is used most commonly to aerosolize medications like pentamidine or to administer intermittent bland aerosol treatments (Fig. 3–7). The output pressure is adjustable up to pressures well above 50 psi, which is useful in controlling flow and, consequently, the amount of aerosol produced. Larger compressors are used to power large volume nebulizers for bland aerosol therapy for tracheostomy and laryngectomy patients (Fig. 3–8).

While very useful, both the tabletop and larger compressors are quite noisy, which may be objectionable for some patients. The tabletop compressor is more noisy and is used only for intermittent treatments. The larger compressor is actually a tabletop compressor in an insulated box that dampens the noise to a more acceptable level. The larger compressor is the equipment of choice for continuous use.

Patient Instruction

The home care RCP teaches the patient to set up the equipment, including proper placement to prevent overheating, and to adjust the operating pres-

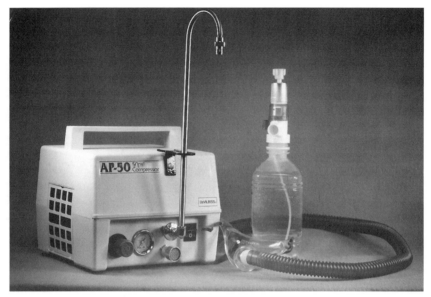

FIGURE 3–8
High-output compressor for continuous aerosol therapy to tracheostomy.

sure, if appropriate. A patient using a tabletop compressor for intermittent aerosol treatment must be shown how to assemble the nebulizer and circuit, which usually consists of large bore tubing; drainage bag; and aerosol mask, tracheostomy mask, or t-piece. If oxygen is being administered with the aerosol, the patient must learn to bleed oxygen into the nebulizer and to adjust the Venturi ring on the large volume nebulizer.

The patient should know how long to take the treatments or when to wear the mask or t-piece and how to time the treatments. The patient must also learn to clean and disinfect the nebulizer and tubing. Nebulizers for either intermittent or continuous use are usually filled with distilled or boiled tap water. Sterile water is expensive and not always covered by insurance, and water straight from the tap contains potentially harmful bacteria.

If a patient is using a tabletop compressor for medication treatments, the home care RCP will teach the patient nebulizer assembly and possibly medication preparation. When pentamidine is being administered, the home care RCP may need to instruct the patient in using a syringe and needle to draw up sterile water or saline from one vial, inject and mix it into a vial of powdered medication, and then withdraw the resultant solution from the vial. Finally, the patient must be advised of proper disposal of syringe, needle, and nebulizer.

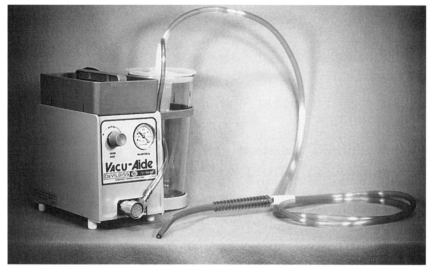

FIGURE 3–9
Home suction machine.

Airway Clearance Devices

Whenever possible, patients should be encouraged to clear their airway by coughing.[8] Patients incapable of adequately clearing their airway by coughing will require mechanical assistance to do so.

Suction Machines

Mechanical airway clearance is most frequently accomplished by using an aspirator, more commonly known as a suction machine. Suction machines are either electricity or battery powered. They are small, easy to operate, and require very little maintenance (Fig. 3–9).

Some patients are able to bring up secretions by coughing but are unable to expectorate the secretions. These patients usually require suctioning of the oropharynx only, using a Yankauer or "tonsil tip" suction handle. Patients with laryngectomies or tracheostomies who are unable to cough will require endotracheal suctioning. Suction catheters are used for endotracheal suctioning. Orotracheal or nasotracheal suctioning is seldom performed at home.

Patients who are entirely dependent on suctioning for airway clearance should have both an electricity- and a battery-powered suction machine in the home to cover the possibility of mechanical failure and power outages. A battery-operated suction machine is also necessary for patients who are away from home and require suctioning.

Patient Instruction.

The home care RCP may have to review coughing techniques with the patient.[8] The home care RCP will also teach the patient and any caregivers the operation of the suction machine and disposal of the suction container's contents by pouring the contents into the toilet. Patients and caregivers will also be taught to clean the suction container, connecting tubing, and suction handle or catheter.

The home care RCP is frequently called on to teach the patient and caregivers to perform the actual suctioning procedure, and it is important for everyone involved to understand the inherent differences in suctioning the patient in the home as opposed to in the hospital.

Patients requiring endotracheal suctioning use the same types of suction catheters that a hospital-based RCP uses. The insertion of the suction catheter into the airway and the suction technique are performed in the same manner as in a hospital. The similarities in endotracheal suctioning diverge regarding the use of the suction catheter. Catheters may be reused repeatedly for several hours in home care, and nonsterile, rather than sterile, gloves are frequently used. Suction catheters are rinsed with boiled water, distilled water, and, in some instances, water straight from the tap. Sterile water is seldom used, is very expensive, and is not paid for by many insurance companies.

Manual Cough Assist Devices

Some patients benefit from the use of manual cough assist devices like the flutter valve, mechanical exsufflation, and positive expiratory pressure (PEP) through a flow resistor.[9] Using the flutter valve, the patient exhales against a resistance, while at the same time a metal ball in the device "flutters," causing high-frequency oscillations in the airway. The mechanical exsufflator gives the patient a positive pressure breath and assists the patient's cough with a negative pressure, causing a rapid, forced exhalation. The PEP device is used to create positive pressure in the airways during a series of breaths that the patient follows with a "huff" cough.

Many patients learn to use these devices in the hospital or by attending specialty clinics (as for cystic fibrosis or muscular dystrophy). Most often the home care RCP will reinforce instructions already given to patients and monitor their technique.

Airway Care

Ancillary procedures such as tracheostomy care and tracheostomy tube maintenance are also taught by the home care RCP,[10] but tracheostomy care is performed somewhat differently in the home than it is in the hospital. Sterile technique is seldom used in the home, and patients may use small bowls to clean the inner cannula and tube rather than a sterile tracheostomy care kit. Some patients clean their inner cannula under running tap water, forgoing the customary half-strength peroxide and boiled water cleaning solution. Although not recommended by the manufacturers, disposable inner cannulas are often cleaned and reused. The tracheostomy stoma is frequently cleaned with soap and water rather than peroxide and water.

Tracheostomy tube changes are done by the patient, the caregivers, the home health nurse, or the home care RCP. Some patients are taken to the physician's office or the Emergency Room for changes, but it is usually much easier to change the tube at home. Family members or other caregivers are frequently taught to change the tracheostomy tube, which is extremely useful when the patient is ventilator-dependent and the tube malfunctions.

Ventilatory Assist Devices

Major advancements in technology for home medical equipment have provided us with the ability to treat many chronic disease states that previously required the patient to remain in the hospital. Ventilatory assist devices are frequently used in home care to treat the long-term needs of patients with chronic respiratory insufficiency, ventilatory failure, or other respiratory problems. Because the focus is on using these devices at home, technology has evolved to make them "user-friendly," allowing home care RCPs to train the lay person to perform many of the duties the RCP and nurse have traditionally performed. This section reviews such ventilatory assist devices as intermittent positive pressure breathing (IPPB) machines and noninvasive and invasive mechanical ventilators, as well as devices to treat sleep-disordered breathing.

Intermittent Positive Pressure Breathing

Although it is not used very often, IPPB is ordered occasionally for the home care patient. IPPB is used most frequently to treat chronic ventilatory insufficiency in patients with neuromuscular disorders like muscular dystrophy and restrictive lung diseases like kyphoscoliosis.[11,12] The home IPPB machine is electricity powered and small enough to sit on a table (Fig. 3–10). Medications may be nebulized during the IPPB treatment.

The main problem with using IPPB at home is that these machines are no longer manufactured. Home care RCPs and patients must contend with using older equipment that may be difficult to repair. The use of this device, however, may delay for a time a patient's need for nocturnal or continuous positive pressure ventilation.

Home Mechanical Ventilation

The most complicated, technical, and time-intensive equipment the home care RCP may set up is a volume ventilator for invasive mechanical ventila-

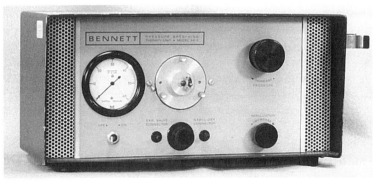

FIGURE 3–10
Intermittent positive pressure breathing (IPPB) machine used in the home.

tion. Home ventilators operate on 110-volt house current but can also run on an external or internal battery. These devices are equipped with alarms to identify high- and low-pressure events or power switchover. They are relatively user-friendly, and patients and caregivers learn to use them very successfully. Home ventilators are fairly lightweight (35 to 40 pounds), which allows them to be portable; many patients have a ventilator mounted to a wheelchair to allow them mobility. Figure 3–11 illustrates a commonly used home ventilator.

The advent of home ventilators has allowed many patients who used to live in a hospital or nursing home to return home. Home ventilator users include both pediatric and adult patients.[13,14] Not every patient who needs long-term invasive mechanical ventilation is a candidate for home ventilator care. A tremendous amount of planning, assessment, and training must take place to prepare a patient for discharge with a ventilator. A complete description of the home mechanical ventilation discharge process is beyond the scope of this book. The reader is urged to consult the bibliography at the end of this chapter as well as review the large volume of printed materials available on this subject.

Noninvasive Home Mechanical Ventilation

Another aspect of home ventilator care is noninvasive mechanical ventilation. This method is used to treat patients with chronic respiratory failure who do not have an artificial airway in place. Noninvasive ventilation is administered via a nasal or full face mask or a chamber device for negative pressure ventilation.

Nasal Positive Pressure Ventilation.

Nasal positive pressure ventilation (NPPV) is applied using a nasal or full face mask or an oral appliance attached to the ventilator circuit. The circuit

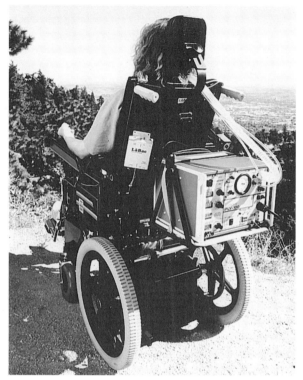

FIGURE 3–11
Commonly used home ventilator. (Courtesy of Respironics, Westminster, CO.)

is connected either to a positive pressure home ventilator or to a continuous flow generator. NPPV is used nocturnally in most patients and has been shown to slow the progression of respiratory insufficiency associated with neuromuscular, obstructive, and restrictive lung diseases.[15-17]

NPPV is difficult for some patients to tolerate at first. The nasal or full face mask is a prime reason for their discomfort. Many patients complain of claustrophobia, facial pain, and headaches from the mask headgear used to hold the mask in place. Good mask fit is essential to NPPV therapy. Many patients have difficulty tolerating the airflow delivered by the ventilator or flow generator, and the volume or pressure may need to be titrated up slowly to allow patients time to adjust to the sensation. It can take several hours or even days to titrate the volume or pressure to the level needed to adequately ventilate the patient. Patience and perseverance are important when applying NPPV.

Negative Pressure Ventilation

Negative pressure ventilation is another method of noninvasive mechanical ventilator support. It is applied using some type of chamber device, such

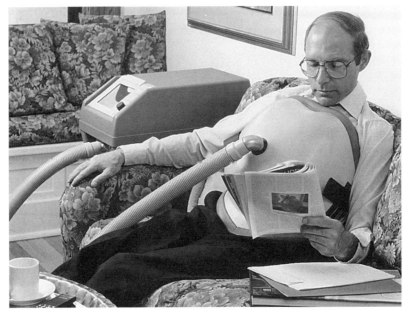

FIGURE 3–12
Negative pressure ventilation by chest shell. (Courtesy of Respironics, Westminster, CO.)

as a chest shell (Fig. 3–12), raincoatlike suit (Fig. 3–13), or iron lung (Fig. 3–14). Negative pressure is applied to the space between the chamber device and the patient's ribcage, causing the chest to rise. Inspiration stops when the preset negative pressure is reached, resulting in a passive exhalation.[18,19]

Negative pressure ventilation is an alternative for the patient who cannot tolerate NPPV. Negative pressure ventilation is difficult to implement, however. The chest shell is bulky and can irritate the patient's skin, and both it and the raincoatlike pneumosuit are difficult to apply, particularly for the patient with muscle weakness. Both are also difficult to seal against leaks. The iron lung is large, heavy, and limited in access for the patient's care procedures. Negative pressure ventilation has also been found to increase the risk of obstructive sleep apnea.[19] Careful patient selection, training, and monitoring, however, can lead to success when using this type of ventilation.

Continuous Positive Airway Pressure/Bilevel Pressure Support Devices

CPAP and bilevel pressure support devices are used to treat a wide array of ventilatory problems. CPAP is most frequently used in the treatment of obstructive sleep apnea and other sleep-related breathing disorders. Bilevel pressure support is also used to treat sleep-related breathing disorders. Bilevel pressure support has been found to be effective as a mode of noninvasive mechanical ventilation in the treatment of acute and chronic respiratory failure.[17,18,20,21]

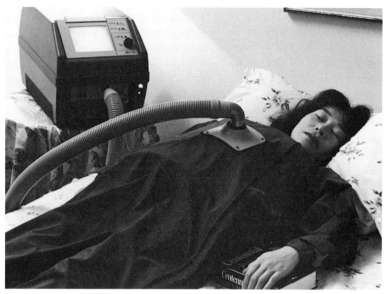

FIGURE 3–13
Negative pressure ventilation by ''pneumosuit.'' (Courtesy of Respironics, Westminster, CO.)

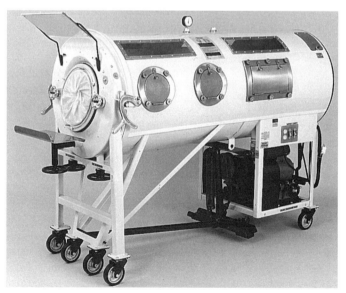

FIGURE 3–14
Iron Lung. (Courtesy of Respironics, Westminster, CO.)

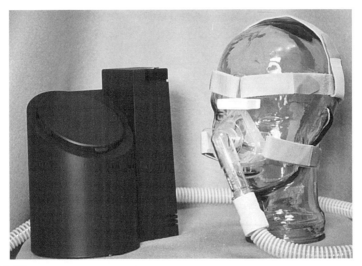

FIGURE 3–15
Home continuous positive airway pressure (CPAP) unit.

The treatment of sleep-related breathing disorders is one of the most rapidly growing segments of home respiratory care. Obstructive sleep apnea (OSA) is being diagnosed with increasing frequency and treated with CPAP and, in some cases, bilevel pressure support. A CPAP device delivers a single preset level of pressure on both inspiration and expiration, and bilevel devices deliver one pressure on inspiration and a lower one on exhalation. Determination of CPAP or bilevel pressure is usually made by the physician based on the results of a sleep study.

Obstructive sleep apnea occurs when the tongue and soft palate drop into the hypopharynx during sleep, partially or completely obstructing the airway. This obstruction prevents the patient from taking a breath. If the obstruction causes prolonged apnea, a drop in oxygen saturation and arrhythmias can occur. These symptoms cause arousal and awakening that can occur hundreds of times during the night while the patient remains unaware. Patients with OSA often spend very little or no time in the deeper levels of sleep and complain of feeling more tired than when they went to bed. Some common signs of OSA are snoring (sometimes obnoxiously loud), moving or jerking of the legs during sleep, thrashing about in bed during sleep, headaches upon awakening, and excessive daytime sleepiness. The related hypoxemia and cardiac and blood pressure irregularities can be potentially life-threatening.[22,23]

CPAP or bilevel therapy works by delivering a pressurized airflow to a nasal mask the patient wears during sleep (Fig. 3–15). This pressurized air acts as a pneumatic splint to prevent the tongue and soft palate from

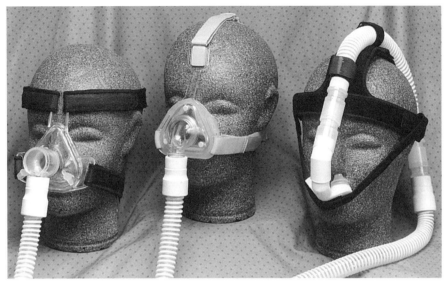

FIGURE 3–16
Different types of CPAP mask applications.

dropping back into the hypopharynx, thereby eliminating the obstruction. CPAP therapy is the most successful method of treating OSA. Other methods, including surgical procedures, nasal strips, and oral appliances have less than satisfactory success rates.[22,23] Figure 3–15 illustrates one type of home CPAP unit.

Bilevel pressure support is frequently being used in the acute care facility as an initial effort to treat respiratory failure in the hope of preventing intubation. Patients with chronic pulmonary diseases who were successfully treated with bilevel pressure support may continue that treatment when discharged home. The home care RCP may also be asked to initiate bilevel pressure support at home for a patient with chronic respiratory disease. In such an instance, pressure levels are set either by specific orders from the physician, or the physician may ask the home care RCP to titrate the pressure levels.

Patient Instruction

CPAP and bilevel pressure support are fairly time-intensive for the home care RCP. As with NPPV, the patient must be properly fitted with a nasal or full face mask that is held in place with headgear. Nasal masks are used far more prevalently than full face masks, although full face masks offer an option for patients who cannot keep their mouths closed during treatment, even when a chin strap is used. Patients who are claustrophobic may find either mask difficult to wear. In this event, the patient may tolerate nasal pillows. Figure 3–16 demonstrates different CPAP mask applications.

TABLE 3–5
COMMON CONTINUOUS POSITIVE AIRWAY PRESSURE PROBLEMS AND SOLUTIONS

Problem	Solution
Pressure sore on face or bridge of nose	Loosen headgear, use spacer cushion on bridge of mask, apply moleskin to affected area, refit with a different size or type of mask.
Dry mouth	Use in-line humidifier, chin strap.
Dry nasal passages, nosebleeds	Use saline nasal spray at bedtime, in-line humidifier.
Nasal stuffiness, sinus irritation, ear pain	Use saline nasal spray, in-line heated humidifier, oral decongestant, nasal decongestant spray, steroid nasal spray.
Cold nose	Place CPAP hose under bedcovers to allow body heat to warm the air, use heated humidifier in-line.
Bothersome machine sound	Place CPAP machine on floor, under bed. Check for leaks, use an extra length of hose, and move the machine away from the bedside.

Once the mask is fit, the patient must then get used to sleeping while wearing it. The patient must also try to fall asleep with a high flow of air going up the nose. Patients with sinus problems may experience an aggravation of these problems. Other patients may experience back problems because they are not used to lying so still during sleep (sleep apnea patients tend to move a great deal with the arousals and awakenings that occur with obstruction). Failure to obtain a seal with the mask results in air leaks around the eyes, causing irritation. Other common problems experienced by CPAP patients are facial sores from the mask, dry nose and mouth, and sometimes nose bleeds. These problems will affect patient compliance if not corrected.[24]

The home care RCP must remain mindful of the difficulties patients can have in adjusting to CPAP or bilevel pressure therapy and try to make the experience as comfortable and easy as possible. Table 3–5 describes common problems and solutions that may help the CPAP patient. Patients and their spouses should also be encouraged to join a CPAP support group.

Diagnostic and Monitoring Devices

Many procedures that previously required a visit to the physician's office, outpatient clinic, or laboratory are now being routinely performed in the home. A patient can have venous and arterial blood samples taken, as well as electrocardiograms and mobile radiographs. The home care RCP is able to perform various types of diagnostic and monitoring procedures to assist in the treatment of the home care patient. These procedures include oximetry,

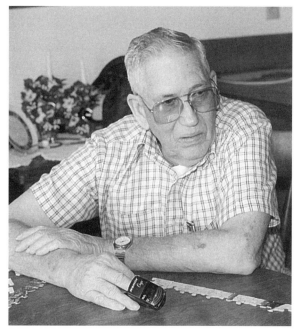

FIGURE 3–17
Portable oximeter.

cardiorespiratory monitoring, basic pulmonary functions, and home sleep studies.

Oximetry

Pulse oximeters are routinely used in the home to monitor SpO_2. Oximeters are used for spot checks as well as for continuous monitoring. Technology has evolved to allow for long-term recording, simultaneous monitoring of several parameters, and exceptional portability (Fig. 3–17). Pulse oximeters are used ideally for periodic measurement of a patient's oxygen saturation levels and to evaluate trends in oxygen saturation during exercise or sleep. Oximetry can help identify changes in lung function and establish the need for a change in or discontinuation of oxygen therapy.

Pulse oximeters present some drawbacks. Oximetry readings can be less than accurate under certain circumstances, and the home care RCP as well as the patient and caregivers must be aware of ways in which inaccurate readings can be obtained. Poor perfusion at the probe site can cause lower than expected readings, which can be a problem in the patient with cold hands or feet or very low blood pressure or with the diabetic patient with poor peripheral perfusion. Warming up the patient's hand or foot before placing the probe will help increase circulation and allow the oximeter to get a better reading in many cases.

Excessive movement of the probe site will also cause inaccurate readings or will prevent the oximeter from reading at all. Elderly patients often have difficulty holding their hands still, and the home care RCP may have to hold the digit still to get a reading. Patients who smoke may have higher than expected results due to carboxyhemoglobin. Studies have shown that dark skin color may give lower oximetry readings, and black, blue, or green nail polish can cause significantly lower readings. Even bright light can interfere with the oximeter's ability to read.[25,26]

The home care RCP must recognize the potential inaccuracies with oximeter readings and take them into account when recommending changes in oxygen therapy. The home care RCP would not necessarily administer supplemental oxygen to a patient whose oximetry reading was low if the reading was difficult to get because the patient had diabetes that caused poor perfusion in the hands. Choosing an alternate site might assist the home care RCP in obtaining more accurate results, allowing him or her to make a better decision regarding the patient's need for supplemental oxygen.

A key issue with oximeter use in the home is the dependence patients and caregivers develop for it. Caregivers will often use oximetry readings alone to identify changes in patient condition rather than look at the entire situation. The patient may experience momentary drops in oxygen saturation that the caregiver may consider significant, when in actuality the patient may have coughed, moved his or her probe site, or needed the probe cleaned. Patients and caregivers should be instructed never to use oximetry results as the only parameter when making care decisions but rather to use those results in the context of the patient's condition.

Some patients become dependent on pulse oximeters in the hospital, where they are more likely to have continuous oxygen saturation monitoring. Adult patients should not require continuous monitoring of SpO_2. The fact that they *are* at home usually indicates that they are stable and not in need of the kind of monitoring they would have in the hospital. Many insurance companies, including Medicare, do not pay for oximeters for home use. Pediatric patients in certain circumstances, such as weaning from a ventilator, may benefit from continuous monitoring by oximetry.[26]

Cardiorespiratory Monitoring

Commonly called *apnea monitors,* these devices are used to monitor heart rate and respiratory frequency and to give an audible alarm when either parameter is outside a preset range. Although occasionally these monitors are used for adults, they most frequently are used for infants. Chapter 4 provides a complete description of this type of monitoring.

Home Sleep Studies

It has been estimated that 37 percent of adults over 60 years of age have obstructive sleep apnea.[23] Patients traditionally go to a sleep laboratory or a sleep disorders center for evaluation and diagnosis, which can involve a 1- to 2-night stay for a comprehensive sleep study. Comprehensive sleep studies may cost several thousands of dollars. As more primary care physicians refer more patients for sleep studies, insurance companies seek less costly alternatives for diagnosing OSA.

An alternative to the comprehensive study that is carried out in a formal sleep laboratory is the home sleep study, and home care RCPs are performing these tests, using small, portable recording devices that monitor parameters such as oxygen saturation, heart rate, airflow, and snoring. The home care RCP delivers the recording device to the patient's home and teaches the patient to attach the monitoring leads (e.g., oximeter probe, microphone, airflow thermistor) and to start and stop the testing. The home care RCP will return the next day to pick up the equipment, download the stored information, and print a hard copy of the night's data. The physician will interpret the data and determine the need for more comprehensive testing or start the patient on CPAP or other therapy.

The home sleep recording device is very useful for screening patients for OSA. A test showing oxygen desaturation during a period of little or no airflow or with exaggerated chest and abdominal movement indicates that OSA may be present. These patients may be referred to a sleep laboratory for a more complete study and for testing while using CPAP. Some physicians believe (and this is echoed by many insurance companies) that the home sleep study is an adequate tool to identify the presence of OSA and will initiate treatment based solely on these results. Once the diagnosis has been made and the physician determines that a trial with CPAP therapy is indicated, the home care RCP may be asked to set up the patient on a starting level of CPAP and titrate the pressure until the patient experiences an improvement in his or her symptoms.

This titration method is controversial because the therapeutic level of CPAP is based on the subjective observations of the patient and input from the patient's sleeping partner, if there is one. Some believe that the only way to determine a patient's therapeutic CPAP level is by conducting an attended multichannel sleep recording while the patient uses a CPAP device, making pressure adjustments during the recording as indicated. Others believe that using a home sleep study as anything more than a screening tool provides for an incomplete diagnosis. It is difficult to argue with success, however, and patients are being evaluated and successfully treated using the results of home sleep studies with increasing frequency, particularly when insurance carriers are viewing the home sleep study as a way to reduce expenditures.

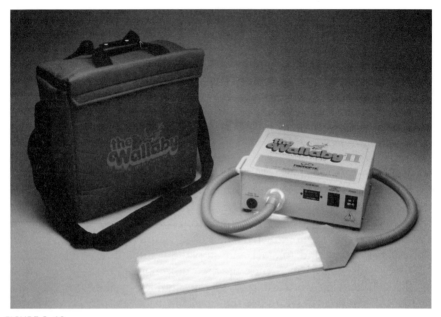

FIGURE 3–18
Phototherapy lights for treatment of hyperbilirubinemia. (Courtesy of Healthdyne Technologies, Marietta, GA.)

Ancillary Home Care Equipment

Home care RCPs are occasionally called on to set up equipment not traditionally used in respiratory care. This is usually because the home care RCP may be the only health care professional employed by the HME/RT company that provides such equipment. Therefore, it is important for the home care RCP to be familiar with the many types of equipment used by home care patients.

Home Phototherapy

Two types of phototherapy are performed in the home. Phototherapy lights for the treatment of hyperbilirubinemia are used for newborns who become jaundiced after birth. A baby needing this treatment either is placed under a bank of special lights or has a panel of fiber-optic lights wrapped around the torso (Fig. 3–18). If overhead lights are used, the baby must remain unclothed and wear eyepatches to protect the eyes. The wrap-around fiber-optic panel allows the baby to be wrapped in a blanket and does not require the use of protective eye covers. The home care RCP will show the parents how to safely use the phototherapy lights, including the prescribed use times. The baby should have daily blood tests to monitor the bilirubin level.

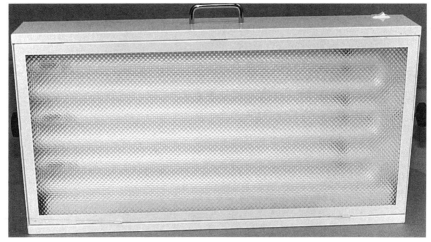

FIGURE 3–19
Phototherapy lights for treatment of sleep disorders like seasonal affective disorder.

Phototherapy lights for the treatment of sleep-related disorders are also used in the home (Fig. 3–19). Problems such as seasonal affective disorder and sleep phase abnormalities can be easily treated with such lights. The physician will order the level of light, the amount of time, and the time of day the patient should use the lights. The home care RCP will show the patient how to set the light level and use the lights as prescribed.

Nutritional Therapy

Some patients, because of a variety of illnesses, are unable to take food or water by mouth. These patients receive nutrition through a feeding tube. RCPs working in the acute care setting are familiar with nasogastric (NG) tubes, but these are not commonly used in the home care setting. Instead, a semipermanent tube known as a gastrostomy or jejunostomy tube is placed through the abdominal wall into the stomach or jejunum. It is through this tube that the patient is fed.

Tube feeding is administered by bolus, gravity, or food pump. Bolus feeding uses a 60-mL syringe with the plunger removed and the syringe connected to the patient's feeding tube. Liquid nutrition is poured into the syringe and allowed to flow into the feeding tube at an uncontrolled rate. Gravity feeding involves using a special bag and tubing set that is hung from an IV pole. The flow of nutrition from the bag to the patient is affected by gravity and depends on the height of the bag. This flow is only somewhat controlled. Patients with nausea, vomiting, and other gastrointestinal problems with bolus or gravity feeding may need a more controlled feeding.

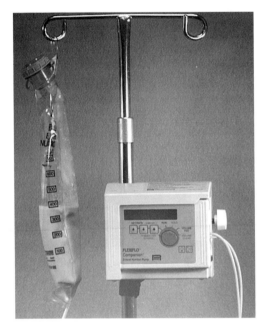

FIGURE 3–20
Enteral therapy pump.

Patients requiring a strictly controlled flow will need an enteral pump, commonly known as a food pump (Fig. 3–20). This controlled flow allows a set volume of nutrition to be administered to the patient via a special bag and tubing set that is attached to the food pump. Most pumps sound an alarm if flow becomes restricted or when all the liquid nutrition has been delivered.

The home care RCP may train the patient and caregivers in the operation of the pump, including how to troubleshoot problems with the pump or pumpset. The home care RCP may also train patients and caregivers in administering gravity feeding. Only properly trained RCPs should perform this type of setup, and the patient and caregivers must understand that problems with the actual feeding tube or stoma site must be referred back to the physician.

IV Therapy

Some home care RCPs set up IV pumps for patients at home. This usually involves teaching the patient and caregivers to set the flow rate and turn the machine on and off and to troubleshoot problems with the pump. A home health nurse works with the patient on the actual medication administration.

TABLE 3–6
**DURABLE MEDICAL EQUIPMENT
COMMONLY PROVIDED BY HOME
MEDICAL EQUIPMENT/RESPIRATORY
THERAPY COMPANIES**

- Hospital beds
- Patient lifts
- Overbed tables
- Overbed trapeze, fracture frames
- Wheelchairs
- Seat lift chairs
- Walkers
- Canes
- Crutches
- Bathroom safety aids
- Commodes
- Bath benches, shower chairs
- Tub transfer benches
- Elevated toilet seats

Glucose Monitors

Home glucose monitoring is very commonly performed by the patient. Home care RCPs often deliver and train patients in the use of glucose monitors. Although relatively simple, the testing procedure, calibration, cleaning, and interpretation of results must be done properly to ensure accurate results. The physician will direct the patient in treating abnormal blood sugar results.

Durable Medical Equipment

Home care RCPs should have a working knowledge of the many types of DME provided by their company. Home care RCPs may be asked to deliver and set up a walker, commode, or wheelchair for a patient they are going to see to eliminate the need for a service technician to deliver it. Home care RCPs may also be asked to evaluate the patient and the environment and to identify areas in which the patient may need assistance. For example, a patient with severe dyspnea may have difficulty walking more than minimal distances and therefore may need a wheelchair. The home care RCP familiar with wheelchairs might recommend a lightweight or electric wheelchair for this patient. A bedside commode may be helpful to this patient if he or she is unable to walk to the bathroom because of dyspnea. A shower chair or hand-held shower attachment may make it easier for the patient to take a shower or bath. Table 3–6 lists types of DME provided by most HME/RT providers.

SUMMARY

This chapter reviews many of the types of home medical equipment home care RCPs may encounter during their workday. As discussed, not all of the equipment is related to respiratory care. The home care RCP must be willing and able to learn to use this equipment and to look at the patient from many different aspects to apply the equipment properly.

The function of the home care RCP is not that of a delivery technician. Although home care RCPs may be delivering equipment, their jobs do not end there. The home care RCP must teach the patient and caregivers the safe and proper use of the equipment, determine whether the environment is appropriate for the equipment (or vice versa), and evaluate the patient for other needs. Most patients require ongoing follow-up while using the home medical equipment and evaluation for changing needs. The RCP who understands the use of both respiratory and nonrespiratory home care equipment is an asset to a company that provides it.

REFERENCES

1. Connors, G and Hilling, L: Definition and overview of pulmonary rehabilitation. In Connors, G and Hilling, L (eds): American Association of Cardiovascular and Pulmonary Rehabilitation: Guidelines for Pulmonary Rehabilitation Programs. Human Kinetics, Champaign, IL, 1993, p 1.
2. Tiep, BL: Long-term home oxygen therapy. Clin Chest Med 3:505, 1990.
3. Hoffman, LA: Novel strategies for delivering oxygen: Reservoir cannula, demand flow, and transtracheal oxygen administration. Respiratory Care 4:363, 1994.
4. O'Donohue, WJ: Transtracheal oxygen: A step beyond the nasal cannula for long-term oxygen therapy. Nebr Med J 11:291, 1992.
5. Wesmiller, SW et al: Exercise tolerance during nasal cannula and transtracheal oxygen delivery. American Review of Respiratory Diseases 141:789, 1990.
6. Oxygen Therapy Guidelines Committee. AARC clinical practice guideline: Oxygen therapy in the home or extended care. Respiratory Care 8:918, 1992.
7. Make, BD: Pulmonary concerns and the exercise prescription. Clin Sports Med 1:105, 1991.
8. Bronchial Hygiene Guidelines Committee. AARC clinical practice guideline: Directed cough. Respiratory Care 5:495, 1993.
9. Hardy, KA and Anderson, BD: Noninvasive clearance of airway secretions. Respiratory Care Clinics of North America 2:323, 1996.
10. Tracheostomy Tube Adult Home Care Guide. Mallinckrodt Medical TPI, Inc., Irvine, CA, 1993.
11. Bach, JR: Pulmonary rehabilitation considerations for Duchenne muscular dystrophy: The prolongation of life by respiratory muscle aids. Critical Reviews in Physical and Rehabilitation Medicine 3:239, 1992.
12. Aerosol Therapy Guidelines Committee. AARC clinical practice guideline: Intermittent positive pressure breathing. Respiratory Care 12:1189, 1993.
13. Gilmartin, M: Transition from the intensive care unit to home: Patient selection and discharge planning. Respiratory Care 5:456, 1994.
14. Kacmarek, RM: Home mechanical ventilatory assistance for infants. Respiratory Care 5:550, 1994.

15. Dean, S and Bach, JR: The use of noninvasive respiratory muscle aids in the management of patients with progressive neuromuscular diseases. Respiratory Care Clinics in North America 2:223, 1996.
16. Leger, P: Long-term noninvasive ventilation for patients with thoracic cage abnormalities. Respiratory Care Clinics of North America 2:242, 1996.
17. Wedzicha, JA: Chronic noninvasive ventilation in obstructive airways disease. Respiratory Care Clinics of North America 2:253, 1996.
18. Hill, NS: Use of negative pressure ventilation, rocking beds, and pneumobelts. Respiratory Care 5:532, 1994.
19. Gilmartin, ME: Body ventilators: Equipment and techniques. Respiratory Care Clinics of North America 2:195, 1996.
20. Waldhorn, RC: Nocturnal nasal intermittent positive pressure ventilation with bi-level positive airway pressure in respiratory failure. Chest 101:516, 1992.
21. Mehta, S and Hill, NS: Noninvasive ventilation in acute respiratory failure. Respiratory Care Clinics of North America 2:267, 1996.
22. Yang, KL: Sleep and sleep-disordered breathing. In Dantzker, DR, MacIntyre, NA and Bakow, EA (eds): Comprehensive Respiratory Care. WB Saunders, Philadelphia, 1995, p 804.
23. Downey, R and Dexter, JR: Assessment of sleep and breathing. In Wilkins, RL, Krider, SJ and Sheldon, RL (eds): Clinical Assessment in Respiratory Care, ed 3. Mosby, St Louis, 1995, p 355.
24. Ordal, KL: Compliance pressure: A CPAP how-to. Journal of Respiratory Care Practitioners 8:57, 1995.
25. Welch, JP, DeCesare, R and Hess, D: Pulse oximetry: Instrumentation and clinical applications. Respiratory Care 6:584, 1990.
26. Kacmarek, RM: Noninvasive monitoring of respiratory function outside of the hospital. Respiratory Care 7:719, 1990.

BIBLIOGRAPHY

Baldwin-Meyers, A et al: Standards of Care for the Ventilator-Assisted Individual: A Comprehensive Management Plan from Hospital to Home. Loma Linda Medical Center, Loma Linda, CA, 1995.

DeWitt, PK et al: Obstacles to discharge of ventilator-assisted children from the hospital to home. Chest 103:1560, 1993.

Gilmartin, ME: Long-term mechanical ventilation: Patient selection and discharge planning. Respiratory Care 36:205, 1991.

Gilmartin, ME and Make, BJ (eds): Mechanical Ventilation in the Home: Issues for Health Care Providers. Problems in Respiratory Care 1:155–295, 1988.

Glenn, KA and Make, BJ: Learning Objectives for Positive Pressure Ventilation in the Home. National Center for Home Mechanical Ventilation and National Jewish Center for Immunology and Respiratory Medicine. Denver, CO, 1993.

Make, BJ et al: Mechanical ventilation beyond the critical care unit: Report of a consensus conference of the American College of Chest Physicians. Chest Oct 1997, in press.

Mizumori, NA et al: Mechanical ventilation in the home. In Turner, J et al: Handbook of Adult and Pediatric Respiratory Home Care. Mosby-Year Book, St Louis, 1994, p 273.

O'Donohue, WJ et al: Long-term mechanical ventilation: Guidelines for management in the home and at alternate community sites. Chest 90:1s, 1986.

Pierson, DJ and Kacmarek, RM: Home ventilator care. In Casaburi, R and Petty, TL (eds): Principles and Practice of Pulmonary Rehabilitation. WB Saunders, Philadelphia, 1993, p 274.

Respiratory Home Care Focus Group: AARC clinical practice guideline: Discharge planning for the respiratory care patient. Respiratory Care 40:1308, 1995.

Respiratory Home Care Focus Group: AARC clinical practice guideline: Long-term invasive mechanical ventilation in the home. Respiratory Care 40:1313, 1995.

chapter 4

Pediatric Respiratory Home Care

Michael McDonald, BS, RRT
Susan L. McInturff, RCP, RRT
Charles McIntyre, RN, RRT

Home respiratory care has become an acceptable and preferred alternative to a hospital stay for children with long-term disorders. Many of today's surviving premature newborns with chronic cardiorespiratory problems will eventually require continued treatment in the home.

The home care industry has undergone rapid growth in this decade, particularly with regard to home respiratory care, especially for the pediatric patient. Technological advances have enabled us to improve survival rates, have made available modalities in home care that were not previously available, and have improved on many procedures that have been in use. This has resulted in the growing need for RCPs with particular knowledge of pediatric respiratory care.

This chapter compares the differences between pediatric home respiratory care and adult home respiratory care. Equipment choices, psychosocial issues, and diagnostic monitoring are discussed. The goal of this chapter is to prepare the RCP to make sound decisions when caring for the pediatric patient at home, bearing in mind that these decisions will likely be different from those made when caring for the adult.

Historical Perspective

In 1963 in the Boston area, an infant was born to a very wealthy and important family. Unfortunately, he was born prematurely at 36 weeks gestation and weighed only 4 lb 10 oz. By today's standards this baby was only slightly premature. His mother had a history of one stillbirth but had also successfully delivered two full-term children who were alive and well. The premature baby, born in a military hospital on Cape Cod, was immediately transferred to Boston Children's Hospital, one of the most forward-thinking infant care centers in the United States at that time.

Thirty-nine hours after birth, the infant died of hyaline membrane disease. Patrick Bouvier Kennedy, son of the sitting President of the United States, could not be saved by the best care available in 1963. Many procedures were attempted to save Patrick Bouvier Kennedy's life. He was soaked in epsom salt solutions. Plasmin was nebulized into his Isolette. Oxygen was used without restriction, but still this infant died after struggling for 39 hours to inflate his lungs with every breath.

Prior to the Middle Ages, premature newborns and infants with congenital deformities were left to die, as little was known about caring for them. During the Middle Ages, humanitarian concerns led to the establishment of homes for these abandoned infants. However, death remained inevitable, and few, if any, of the infants survived. Technological development of the first incubation system by a group of French physicians in the 19th century led to a striking improvement in survival rates and establishment of the first newborn care center in Paris.[1]

In 1900 the newborn mortality rate was approximately 100 per 1000 live births.[2] This rate declined steadily throughout the first half of the decade to 20 per 1000 live births by 1950.[1] By 1975 the number dropped to 11.6 per 1000.[2] Survival rates for these infants have steadily improved over the years to include a higher percentage of infants weighing less than 2500 g, with an appreciable percentage of those babies weighing less than 1500 g at birth.

Major discoveries and improvements have been made in the field of neonatology and pediatrics since the 1960s. The development of positive

RDS & hyaline membrane disease

pressure ventilation, intermittent mandatory ventilation (IMV), and continuous positive airway pressure (CPAP) gave us treatment options that were not available before. These methodologies were successfully supported by the rapid development of accurate, simplified techniques for blood gas determinations. These developments have been paramount to the success of treating pathologies such as respiratory distress syndrome and hyaline membrane disease. Neonatology and respiratory care have developed rapidly together in the last 25 years. Such changes have also occurred in home care.

Relative Costs: Home versus Hospital

Infants who are ill from birth or who develop a chronic disease process are traditionally cared for in the acute care hospital, very often in a pediatric intensive care unit. The cost of care of these infants is one of the most expensive of all types of hospitalizations. Many technology-dependent children remain in acute care facilities for long periods, even though they are considered to be medically stable.[3] As hospital costs for the care of these stable patients threaten to reach catastrophic levels, the alternative of home care must be considered. This is particularly important, given today's cost consciousness by insurance companies.

Consider hospital costs for a ventilator-dependent pediatric patient, estimated to exceed $2000 per day.[3] The cost of purchasing the equipment needed to care for the child at home is estimated to be equivalent to the cost of keeping the child in an intensive care unit (ICU) for only a few days.[4] The major impediment to sending technology-dependent children home, however, is the lack of funding.[5] As hospitals and insurance companies see the financial value of sending these types of patients home, funding becomes more accessible.

The Pediatric Patient

Some major differences in anatomy, physiology, and development characterize the pediatric patient. Although the home care RCP will not be working with unstable neonates but rather with stable infants, it is important to be aware of these differences to know how they can affect the patient's respiratory status. This knowledge can aid the home care RCP in identifying problems (or nonproblems, as the case may be) that may be assessed during the home visit.

For clarity, it is helpful to differentiate the pediatric patient by age[6]:

- Gestational age: the age of the infant computed from the date of conception

- Chronological age: the age of the infant computed from the date of birth
- Preterm infant: born at 37 weeks or less of gestational age
- Term infant: born between 38 and 42 weeks of gestational age
- Postterm infant: born at 43 or more weeks of gestational age
- Young infant: less than 3 months old
- Older infant: between 3 and 12 months old
- Child: between 12 months and adolescence

Anatomical Differences

There are several anatomical differences in the infant's respiratory system versus the adult's. Infants tend to naturally breathe through their noses, and it is estimated that the nasal passages provide approximately 50 percent of the total resistance to respiration.[7] The soft palate is much greater in size, and the adenoids are larger, decreasing in size as the child grows older. The eustachian tubes are relatively horizontal, allowing fluid to back up into the middle ear much more readily and not allowing fluid to drain easily.

The larynx is located two to three cervical vertebrae higher in an infant, which makes the infant more vulnerable to aspiration. The airways have smaller lumens, and the proportion of soft tissue and mucus-producing glands is greater in the infant. The infant's cricoid cartilage is much smaller than an adult's. These factors significantly increase the risk of airway obstruction.

There is less cartilaginous support of the small airway, making the infant's airways more prone to collapse. The airways are also more prone to spasm. The pores of Kohn, the channels between the alveoli that allow for collateral ventilation, are thought to be nonfunctional at birth but develop as the infant grows. Atelectasis is a real concern when these factors are considered.

The infant's thoracic cage is also different. At birth the sternum is cartilaginous and quite soft. The ribs are also soft and do not provide much support. The diaphragmatic excursion and "bucket-handle" movement of the rib cage does not occur in the infant as it does in the adult.

Physiological Differences

The normal heart rate for an infant is 100 to 160 beats per min (bpm). A pulse rate higher than 160 is considered tachycardic and can be caused by crying, pain, or increased body temperature (above 37.5°C). Bradycardia can occur when hypoxia is present, when body temperature is decreased (less than 36°C), and when the infant cries vigorously. The normal heart rate slows as the infant becomes older.[6]

An infant's respiratory rate is much faster than an adult's. A normal

TABLE 4–1
**CHRONIC RESPIRATORY DISEASES
COMMONLY SEEN IN HOME CARE**

- Bronchopulmonary dysplasia (BPD)
- Cystic fibrosis
- Asthma
- Congenital central hypoventilation syndrome (Ondine's curse)
- Werdnig-Hoffmann disease
- Bronchomalacia
- Tracheomalacia
- Tracheal stenosis
- Arnold-Chiari deformity
- Trisomy 13
- Gastroesophageal reflux
- Muscular dystrophy
- Apnea of prematurity

respiratory rate for an infant is between 30 and 60 bpm; this of course decreases as the child becomes older. The infant's respiratory rate can increase in response to pain, anxiety, hypoxemia, hyperthermia, or crying. This increased respiratory rate is called tachypnea.

The normal PaO_2 for an infant is similar to that of an adult: 60 to 100 mm Hg. In general, arterial PaO_2 values of 55 mm Hg and below or oxygen saturations by pulse oximetry of less than 90 percent indicate the need for supplemental oxygen therapy in infants. The deleterious effects of hypoxemia are well documented. Studies have shown that inappropriate discontinuation of home oxygen therapy in infants with bronchopulmonary dysplasia resulted in growth retardation and weight loss.[8]

It is important to remember that the PaO_2 can alter very rapidly in an infant; even normal activities such as crying can cause a drop in the infant's arterial oxygen level. The RCP must be aware of this possibility, because a seemingly small change can become a life-threatening situation for an infant if not corrected immediately.

Chronic Pediatric Respiratory Diseases

There are many diseases common to the pediatric patient that the RCP will assist in treating at home. Many of these diseases have been treated in the critical state while the infant or child was hospitalized and have moved into the chronic state. Some will cause the pediatric patient lifelong problems; others will eventually be outgrown. Table 4–1 lists some of the chronic disease states treated at home.

TABLE 4–2
**SIGNS OF STRESS AND POOR COPING
THAT MAY BE IDENTIFIED DURING
THE PEDIATRIC HOME VISIT**

- Unusual misbehavior by the child
- Displaced anger by the child or the parent
- Hostility from the child or the parent
- Noncompliance from the child or the parent
- Unusual dependency by the child or the parent
- Unusual avoidance or withdrawal by the child

Psychosocial Issues

It is hard to imagine the psychological impact of having a child with a serious illness. Compound that by having a child with a serious illness who requires continuous assisted ventilation, suctioning, tracheostomy tube changes, breathing treatments, tube feedings, diaper changes, physical therapy, and myriad other procedures. The burden may appear to be unbearable, yet this is asked of parents of technology-dependent children.

One of the most serious issues that must be faced is the grief of the parents. Parents of a seriously ill newborn may grieve for the baby they imagined and expected after months of anticipation. In the case of a chronically ill child, the grief is for the loss of what was and for what could have been. The family that is finally bringing home its sick child may continue to grieve while absorbing the extra work involved in caring for the child as well as caring for the other children and their household.

The goals of pediatric home care are to allow the child to function at the highest possible level within a nurturing home environment.[9,10] Older children are encouraged to attend school, and even infants and younger children are started in special out-of-the-home schooling as soon as possible. The strain on the family can be heavy, however. Some parents become overprotective of the child, focusing on the disease rather than the child.[9] These parents, by providing so much attention to the child, may prevent that child from developing properly and learning from his or her experiences. They may have lower expectations for the child, which moves the child further from normal development.

Other parents may deny the reality of the child's illness, in essence rejecting the child. These parents may focus their attentions more on the child's siblings. They may have expectations of their sick child that are unrealistic. In extreme circumstances the parents may abandon the child.

It is important for the RCP to be able to identify emergent psychosocial issues during home visits and report any significant findings to the physician. Table 4–2 lists identifiable signs of stress and poor coping.

The Role of the Respiratory Care Practitioner in Pediatric Home Care

The differences in the anatomy, physiology, and psychosocial aspects of the pediatric patient require the skills of an RCP familiar with neonatal and pediatric respiratory care. The rules that are applied to the care of the adult patient do not necessarily apply to infants or children. That is precisely the reason not every home medical equipment (HME) provider is capable of managing the pediatric patient. Facilities that are planning to discharge a technology-dependent pediatric patient should seek an HME provider that employs a clinician specializing in this type of care.

Requisite Skills

Any RCP practicing home care must have highly developed assessment skills. Any RCP practicing pediatric home care must have the same abilities for assessment but must be able to apply those skills to the pediatric patient. Ideally, the pediatric home care RCP will not only have honed his or her skills by working in an acute care facility but will also have specialized in pediatric acute care. Working at a children's hospital is a good way to develop an understanding of pediatric physiology. Working at a general hospital that has an active neonatal intensive care unit (NICU) or pediatric intensive care unit (PICU) is also useful.

The RCP must have a clear understanding of the differences between pediatric patients and adults and must be able to accurately perform a physical assessment on that pediatric patient. The RCP should also understand the pathophysiology of common respiratory diseases of childhood and the appearance of these diseases in the chronic states.

Moreover, the RCP must feel comfortable working with babies and children, and not every clinician is able to do this. Families are looking for an RCP who is confident, sympathetic, and competent. Parents and, especially, the child may detect that the RCP is uncertain or uncomfortable, and this only adds to the stress the family already feels.

The Respiratory Care Practitioner as Educator

The single most important role of the pediatric home care therapist is as a teacher. The home care RCP is responsible for teaching all the caregivers to properly operate and maintain the equipment being used and for assessing the child's environment for changes that may be necessary to improve the ultimate outcomes of care. This may be as simple as identifying any triggers for asthma that are observed, accompanied by a clear explanation of the reasons for suggested changes. It could also be by setting up a ventilator on a wheelchair to allow the child to go to school.

TABLE 4–3
**SAMPLE TEACHING PROCEDURE FOR PATIENTS,
PARENTS, AND OTHER CAREGIVERS**

1. Explain and review written materials. Materials should be written in terms easily understood by the lay person. Materials should be left with the family for future reference.
2. Provide deliberate and careful demonstration of the skill.
3. Request a return demonstration with verbal recant by the learner of the steps as well as the rationale for those steps in the process. This technique would be supplemented by additional instruction or correction by the instructor.
4. Request another return demonstration, repeated as necessary, with no interruption from the instructor. This reinforcement demonstrates to both the learner and the instructor that the skill is understood and can be performed properly.

Teaching parents and other caregivers to perform care procedures requires an understanding of how people learn. For example, some people are visual learners and learn best from reading flip charts, watching videos, or reading written instructions. Others are auditory learners, learning more easily by listening to lectures, group discussions, or audiotapes. Manual skills are most easily learned and retained through physical demonstration of those skills. The best method for teaching most people is to include all of these aspects. Table 4–3 outlines a sample procedure for teaching the home care patient or caregivers. Regardless of the equipment or procedures being taught, the RCP must be sure that understanding and competency have been achieved.

It is critical to transfer the confidence that the parents have developed in their own abilities during the training session to actual performance with their child. It is also critical to transfer the confidence the child has in the hospital staff to the parents. Many parents anticipate that they will be unable to perform the care for their child as well as the medical professionals in the hospital. Everyone on the health care team, including the parents and the patient, should feel that the child will be safely and properly cared for at home. Having the parents practice all care procedures repeatedly until they can perform them confidently will ensure this.

The Home Visit

Pediatric respiratory home care patients often require close follow-up because of the rapid changes that occur with their growth and development. This is accomplished by periodic visits to the home, supplemented with telephone follow-up. The frequency of follow-up is determined by the child's needs and level of required care. For example, a child who is using a compressor-nebulizer for bronchodilator treatments may require only a follow-up by telephone to determine whether the parents are able to give the child the treatments as prescribed. During the telephone call, the RCP may deter-

TABLE 4–4
ELEMENTS OF THE HOME VISIT

- Interview patient (if possible) and parents or other caregivers to determine current status.
- Evaluate response to treatment.
- Identify problems.
- Make physical assessment.
- Assess environment.
- Evaluate cleaning and maintenance procedures.
- Reinstruct as indicated.
- Involve parents in plan for next follow-up.
- Report all findings to physician.

mine that the parents are uncertain about cleaning and disinfecting the nebulizer or are confused about the timing of the treatments. The RCP may decide to schedule a home visit to reinstruct the parents on these procedures. Another telephone follow-up may determine that the parents are using and maintaining the nebulizer appropriately and do not require further follow-up.

The technology-dependent child generally requires more frequent and ongoing follow-up. This patient may be seen daily for the first several days after discharge to ensure that the equipment is meeting the patient's needs and that the parents and other caregivers are able to manage the care. Knowing that the home care RCP is going to be a frequent visitor goes a long way to reassure parents. Once the family has settled in and is managing the equipment and care satisfactorily, the home visits might be reduced to once a week for the first month, then once every 2 weeks for the next month. A monthly visit may be all that is required for the long-term follow-up of the child and family, unless there is a change in the patient's status. Such changes require a change in the follow-up plan.

The home visit should contain the same elements of assessment that are performed on the adult. Table 4–4 reviews the elements of the home visit. The home visit should be used to compare the child's current status with future expectations. Whether the child is using only a compressor-nebulizer, requires a home ventilator, or is at a level of care in between, the RCP must carefully assess the child's and the family's needs and develop an appropriate follow-up schedule.

The RCP should always attempt to schedule the home visit in advance. Parents may feel they are being checked on if the RCP makes an unannounced visit. The RCP becomes an invited guest in the home and must respect this.

Working with parents in the home also requires a different relationship than that cultivated in the hospital setting. During the hospital stay the parents have turned over much of the decision-making process to the hospital staff. Once at home the parents must become the decision makers. The professional staff must step back and allow them to make these decisions regarding their child's care; the role of the RCP and other professionals at this point is to help the parents by giving them all the information and assistance they need to make proper decisions.

Equipment Used for Pediatric Respiratory Home Care

Some of the types of home respiratory care equipment used for the pediatric patient are designed specifically for the smaller size of this patient. However, many of the types of home respiratory care equipment used for the pediatric patient are also used on adults. It is important for the RCP to understand how to properly use the equipment dependent on the type of patient using it.

Nebulizer Therapy

The type of pediatric patient seen most frequently in the home is the child requiring bronchodilator therapy by compressor-nebulizer, although many pediatric patients are also successfully treated with metered-dose inhalers.[11] The need for bronchodilator therapy tends to be seasonal, just as it is in the acute care setting. Children tend to come down with colds, flu, bronchitis, or an exacerbation of asthma during the winter months and allergy problems during the spring, summer, and fall.

Bronchodilator treatments are given with the same compressor-nebu- lizer as is used by adults. The primary difference is the way in which the medication nebulizer is used. Infants and very young children may be incapable of putting the nebulizer's mouthpiece into their mouth or keeping it there. When setting up a compressor-nebulizer for these children, the parents are usually taught to point the nebulizer toward the nose and mouth of the child (Fig. 4–1). They may have to follow the child's face as the child tries to avoid the aerosolized medication. Another method is to remove the "tee" entirely from the nebulizer and hold the nebulizer below the child's face, allowing the aerosol to flow up past the nose and mouth. Pediatric aerosol masks can be used, but most small children will not tolerate the mask's being strapped to the face.

Small children often salivate copiously during the treatment if they chew on the mouthpiece or hold it in their mouth. Because saliva can run down into the nebulizer, vigorous rinsing of the nebulizer after treatment is advisable to prevent clogging of the nebulizer jet.

Parents should be instructed not to terminate the treatment before all the medication is nebulized. This can be difficult when the child becomes tired of sitting still. It is helpful to distract the child during the treatment. Allowing the child to watch cartoons or a video is a good way to do this.

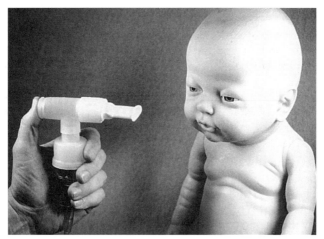

FIGURE 4–1
Administration of nebulizer treatment to an infant.

It is also important for the parents to administer around-the-clock treatments if such treatments have been ordered by the physician. These orders frequently are given during the first 24 or 48 hours of bronchodilator therapy.

Some children will take their compressor-nebulizers to their school or daycare. The RCP may be called on to instruct the day-care providers and school teachers in the use of the nebulizer as well as about signs and symptoms the child may exhibit indicating the need for a treatment.

Oxygen Therapy Devices

The intelligent and careful administration of oxygen to infants has dramatically improved their survivability. Critically ill infants who required extremely high doses of oxygen while in the NICU may finally be discharged from the hospital. These infants have been weaned down to a much lower oxygen concentration, sometimes even to a fraction of a liter. As with any type of oxygen therapy, the goal is to use the lowest oxygen concentration possible to keep the PaO_2 at an acceptable level. Oxygen toxicity in neonates is well known to RCPs, with its resultant interstitial fibrosis, hyperplasia, and pulmonary fibrosis.[12] There is very little risk of toxicity occurring in the home, and the home care RCP will more likely be treating the baby at home who is recovering from the effects of oxygen toxicity. The home care RCP should remain mindful of it, nonetheless.

Delivery Techniques

The equipment used to deliver oxygen therapy to children at home is the same as that used for adults: the liquid oxygen (LOX) system, high-pressure oxygen cylinders, and the oxygen concentrator. (Consult Chapter 3 of this book for a review of these systems.) The system that is chosen depends on the child's needs and oxygen flow rate. There will be times when the child needs oxygen at 1 L/min or more. An oxygen concentrator might be the system of choice for this patient. For oxygen flows of ¼ to 1 L/min or higher, a LOX system is usually the system of choice, particularly when the child needs portability. Higher oxygen flows (greater than 6 L/min) are most easily achieved with a LOX system equipped with a flow controller that is capable of providing those flows.

What is the equipment of choice when the child has been receiving oxygen via an oxygen blender at the hospital? An oxygen blender is not feasible in the home because of the amount of equipment needed for power. It would require not only a large volume 50-psi oxygen source, but a large volume 50-psi compressed gas source as well. There are much easier ways to provide a comparable F_{IO_2} to the child. A standard technique used in home oxygen delivery is to use a very low flow rate of 100 percent oxygen to deliver the proper amount. This is achieved primarily through trial and error, adjusting the flow rate and monitoring the child's oxygen saturation. Many times this conversion results in very low flow rates, sometimes as low as 1/32 of a liter or less, requiring the use of a special flowmeter that is calibrated to deliver such low flow rates.

When very low flow rates are used, the choice of delivery systems is very limited. Liquid oxygen is generally not used at flow rates of less than ¼ L/min because the normal evaporative loss of the LOX tank would be greater than the amount actually used by the patient. Oxygen concentrators are not often used at these low flows because, although there are models calibrated to deliver such flow rates, the cost of the equipment is much greater than its alternatives. The system of choice would be a small compressed oxygen cylinder. For example, a child using a flow rate of 1/32 L/min continuously would use an E tank, which at this flow rate would last 2 weeks. This tank could also serve as the child's portable system, or an even smaller tank such as the M6 size could be used for portability.

Delivery Devices

The types of devices used to administer oxygen in the home are the same as those used in the hospital, with a few exceptions.[13] The nasal cannula is the delivery device used most frequently, and cannulas are now made to fit children, infants, and even premature infants of very small size (Fig. 4–2).

Use of the nasal cannula in infants and children can present some difficulties. One of the most frequently encountered problems is the infant or child who will not leave the cannula in the nose. Using paper or plastic surgical tape to secure the cannula to the child's cheeks is a good way to

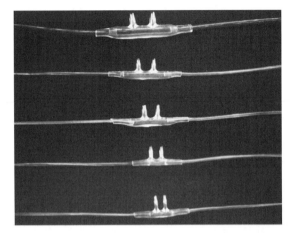

FIGURE 4–2
Comparison of nasal cannula sizes. (*Top*) Cannula for the pediatric patient. (*Bottom*) Cannula for the neonatal patient.

keep the cannula in the nose, but as the child grows older he or she may learn to remove it, despite efforts to prevent it.

One alternative is to use a nasopharyngeal catheter. This is a method seldom used for adults but commonly used with infants. This delivery method uses a very small catheter that is carefully inserted into the nostril and advanced only as far as the nasopharynx. The other end of the catheter is routed out of the end of the nostril and up along the cheek, coming to rest over the ear. The catheter must be secured to the baby's face with tape. For the persistent child, the oxygen tubing can also be affixed to the back of the neck. It is recommended that the catheter be alternated between nares every 8 to 12 hours and changed daily.[13] Use of the nasal catheter is helpful when the child is likely to remain on oxygen for an extended time and continuous observation cannot be provided.

Although several sizes of nasal cannulas are commercially available, there are times when no one size fits the patient just right. For such a patient, the nasal cannula can be modified by cutting off the prongs and cutting an opening between the resultant holes (Fig. 4–3). The tubing must be taped to the cheek as with the conventional cannula.

Evaluation of Oxygen Needs

Children have an advantage over adults in that, as they grow, they are also growing healthy lung tissue. The new lung tissue allows them to overcome some of the damage caused by such diseases as bronchopulmonary dysplasia (BPD) and pneumonia.[7] Consequently, a pediatric patient's oxygen requirements can be expected to change. For this reason, periodic evaluation of the

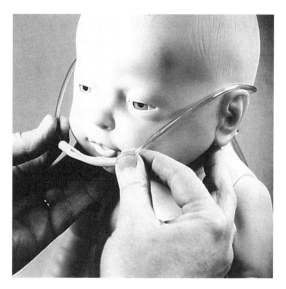

FIGURE 4–3
Cannula modified by cutting off prongs and cutting an opening between the resultant holes.

minimum required oxygen flow is essential to the management of pediatric patients as they grow.

An objective, reviewable method of determining oxygen flow requirements for a child at specific moments can be provided by a state-change study. This is a 3- to 4-hour attended study during which the child's oxygen saturation is monitored through multiple changes of state, from awake and active to quietly asleep. It includes periods of feeding and active play. The RCP will vary the oxygen flow during these states to maintain the oxygen saturation at the level that has been determined appropriate by the physician. Many physicians feel that the pediatric patient's oxygen saturation should remain above 95 percent during all states.[14]

Cardiorespiratory Monitoring

In 1972, it was reported that two of five infants with documented prolonged apnea died of sudden infant death syndrome (SIDS).[15] Since then, much attention has been focused on the relationship between apnea and SIDS. This relationship prompted the development of cardiorespiratory monitors designed for home use. Cardiorespiratory monitoring devices alert parents or caregivers to abnormally long pauses in breathing or marked changes in heart rate, allowing for appropriate intervention in potentially life-threatening situations. Following the passage of the Sudden Infant Death Syndrome Act of 1974, research and clinical programs were mandated that generated reports about apnea, SIDS, and the use of home monitoring devices.[15] Since that time, home monitoring has grown to become an elemental part of the care of at-risk infants. Secondary to compressor-nebulizers, this type of equipment is set up most frequently by the home care RCP.

Types of Apnea

Apnea is classically defined as a cessation of ventilatory airflow.[16] This interruption of ventilation can be either central or obstructive in origin. *Central* apnea is caused by an abnormality in the control mechanism of the medullary respiratory centers of the brain. This abnormality causes an absence of ventilatory effort, causing an absence of airflow.[16]

Obstructive apnea occurs when the upper airway becomes occluded, causing an absence of airflow despite continued ventilatory effort.[16] This may be the result of anatomical, structural, or mechanical abnormalities of the upper airway. The combination of central and obstructive apneas is referred to as *mixed* apnea.

The clinical significance of apnea is determined by the duration of the event and whether it is accompanied by other clinically monitored or observed events. Pathological apnea is defined as a respiratory pause of 20 sec or longer with cyanosis, marked pallor or hypotonia, or bradycardia (less than 100 bpm in infants).[15] However, it is generally accepted that the same event is significant when it lasts 15 sec.[16]

At-Risk Infants

Home monitoring of selected infants appears to be effective in preventing death due to apnea.[17] Cardiorespiratory monitors are generally prescribed for several populations of at-risk infants.

Apnea of Prematurity

Periodic breathing is a condition commonly seen in preterm as well as in some term infants.[17] Periodic breathing is characterized by pauses in ventilation of greater than 3 sec but not long enough to be classified as apnea. When periodic breathing occurs with pathological apnea in the premature newborn, it is referred to as *apnea of prematurity (AOP)*.[15,16] Approximately half of all infants of less than 28 weeks gestation who manifest periodic breathing will have AOP.[16]

AOP generally resolves by 36 weeks postconceptual age, but periodic breathing may persist up to 3 months postterm.

Apnea of Infancy

Term infants (greater than 37 weeks gestation) may also have pathological apnea, referred to as *apnea of infancy (AOI)*. AOI is often unexplained unless known etiologies can be determined. Some of the more common causes of

TABLE 4–5
INDICATIONS FOR HOME MONITORING*

- History of ALTEs requiring vigorous stimulation or resuscitation
- Sibling of two or more SIDS victims

Considerations for home monitoring:
- Infants with less severe ALTEs
- Sibling or twin of a SIDS victim
- Infants with tracheostomies
- Infants of drug-abusing mothers

*This table is not representative of all conditions that may warrant monitoring, but it does include all general conditions constituting high risk for sudden death.
Source: Adapted from the NIH Consensus Statement on Infantile Apnea and Home Monitoring, Sept 1986.[15]

AOI are sepsis, anemia, seizure disorders, hypothermia, and gastroesophageal reflux.[16,18]

Apparent Life-Threatening Event

Any of the previously mentioned conditions may precipitate an *apparent life-threatening event (ALTE)*. An ALTE is defined as an episodic event characterized by a combination of apnea, color change, loss of muscle tone, and choking or gagging.[17] These events may often result in resuscitation attempts and are often confused with SIDS or "near miss" SIDS. It should be noted that an ALTE describes a clinical syndrome with an identifiable cause, whereas SIDS is the sudden death of an infant or child that is unexplained by history or postmortem examination.[18]

If a history and physical examination determines that this episode deserves to be designated an ALTE, the infant will be evaluated for a treatable illness, such as infection or anemia. Once the illness is treated, the child does not require cardiorespiratory monitoring. Other ALTEs have no discernible cause, and it is for these children that home monitoring is considered.

Home Monitoring   alert system for

The decision to monitor an infant or child at home is based on the severity of risk for sudden death. The two groups at highest risk are those with a history of one or more ALTEs requiring vigorous stimulation or resuscitative measures and the siblings of two or more SIDS victims.[15,16] The decision for home monitoring is weighed by the potential benefits as well as the psychosocial burdens placed on the family. It is important that the family understand that using an apnea monitor does not guarantee the survival of the infant and will not prevent ALTEs from occurring.

Cardiorespiratory monitoring is not indicated for normal infants, nor is routine monitoring of preterm infants warranted.[15] Table 4–5 lists indications and considerations for home monitoring.

monitor apnea, bradycardia, tachycardia, et Sat O_2

Home Monitoring Devices

The primary purpose of a home monitor is to detect cardiorespiratory problems so that intervention can take place. The monitor also serves the secondary purpose of providing important information to the physician with regard to frequency, duration, and severity of events.

Cardiorespiratory monitors are small, lightweight, electrically powered devices that use impedance pneumography. This principle is based on changes in resistance that occur during inspiration and expiration. As the lungs expand with air, the impedance to the electrical signal to the infant's chest causes the monitor to increase the electrical energy required to complete the circuit between electrodes placed on the chest. The monitor senses the increase in electrical energy and interprets it as a respiration. The electrodes also pick up the changes in electrical signals associated with the beating of the heart.

The electrodes used during cardiorespiratory monitoring are either rubber or the stick-on type seen in the hospital. The electrodes are placed under each arm at midaxillary nipple level (Fig. 4–4). The rubber electrodes are held in place by an expandable belt. The electrodes are attached to lead wires which, in turn, are connected to a cable that transmits the electrical signals to the monitor.

The cardiorespiratory monitor uses set parameters to detect apneic, bradycardiac, and tachycardiac events. These parameters are ordered by the physician and set by the RCP prior to initial placement on the infant. Typical apnea intervals are set to alarm if no ventilatory effort is made within 10 to 30 sec. Low heart rate alarms can be set from 40 to 100 bpm, and high heart rates range from 150 to 300 bpm, depending on the manufacturer. Settings are determined based on the age and medical status of the infant. When parameters are violated the monitor will emit a loud beeping sound.

Monitor alarms serve not only as a means of alerting the parents to specific events but also as an audible stimulant that often prompts the infant to take a breath, thus interrupting an apneic or related event. This interruption may silence the alarm before the caregiver can respond, leaving the caregiver to wonder what happened. Today's cardiorespiratory monitors have visual indicators that remain lit to identify the alarm; the indicator light can be turned off by activating a reset button. There are also audible alarms and visual indicators to indicate poor connections, faulty electrodes or lead wires, or cable and intrinsic monitor malfunction. Equipment alarms are audibly different from human alarms in that equipment alarms emit a continuous sound, while human alarms make a beeping sound to indicate a change in heart rate or breathing outside the set parameters. Today's monitors also have certain steps that must be taken to turn the monitors off. These so-called sibling alarms prevent the monitor from being turned off accidentally by a child or other unauthorized person.

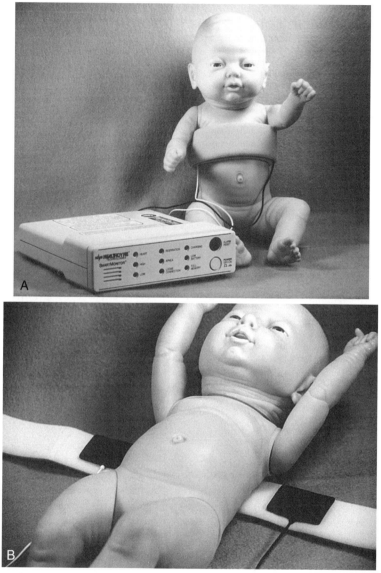

FIGURE 4–4
(*A*) One type of apnea monitor. (*B*) Proper electrode placement for apnea monitoring.

TABLE 4–6
TROUBLESHOOTING TECHNIQUES FOR HOME APNEA MONITORS

Determine whether the audible alarm is beeping, denoting a human alarm, or a constant tone, denoting an equipment alarm.

If the alarm is beeping:

1. Go to the baby.
2. If the alarm has stopped, identify which one it was by seeing which alarm light remains lit. Observe the baby. If the baby is breathing and does not appear to be in any distress, record the alarm on the event log.
3. If the alarm has not stopped, identify which alarm is lit: apnea, bradycardia, tachycardia, or a combination. Observe the baby for breathing, color change, loss of muscle tone, gagging, or choking.
4. If the baby is breathing and appears to be in no distress, check the placement of the electrodes and the position of the electrode belt. Reposition or replace electrodes.
5. If the baby is breathing but is difficult to arouse, stimulate by flicking the cheek or bottoms of the feet, or pick the baby up.
6. If the baby is not breathing, call 911 and begin CPR.

If the alarm is continuous, denoting an equipment problem:

1. Go to the baby.
2. Identify the equipment alarm: loose connection, low battery, full memory, monitor failure.
3. If no alarm lights are lit, check to see if someone has tried to turn the monitor off without following the proper sequence.
4. If there is a loose connection alarm, check the position and fit of the electrode belt. Tighten or reposition it as necessary.
5. Clean the surface of the rubber electrodes and rub a few drops of tap water onto their surfaces to increase conductivity. Replace stick-on electrodes as necessary.
6. Replace lead wires if previous steps do not correct alarm.
7. Plug monitor into electricity if the battery is low.
8. Contact the HME provider if the memory is full.
9. Contact the HME provider if attempts to correct an equipment alarm are unsuccessful.

Today's apnea monitors are equipped with internal batteries that allow the monitors to be used away from an AC power source for up to several days. Many are also equipped with the capability of recording and storing events, including human and equipment alarms and use times.

Training Parents and Caregivers

An essential element to the proper use of a cardiorespiratory monitor in the home is thorough training of all persons who will be responsible for using it. The training should include how and when to use the monitor, proper response to alarms, and care and cleaning of electrodes. The parents must also be capable of troubleshooting the alarms; Table 4–6 outlines steps to be taken in troubleshooting alarms.

Parents should always be taught to perform infant cardiopulmonary resuscitation *before* taking the baby home. This training can be provided by the hospital staff or by the home care RCP who is certified as a cardiopulmonary resuscitation (CPR) instructor.

Documented Monitoring

Parents are taught to record alarm events as they occur using an "event log." This log provides details of the events and actions required by the parents to correct the alarms. The information is used to identify trends in alarms (such as when they occur regularly after feedings or during deep sleep) and can help the physician determine appropriate treatment. A problem with these event logs is that some parents do not keep them. Another common problem is that the family may be noncompliant with monitor use.

This lack of objective documentation has led to the development of recording or "memory" monitors. These monitors are programmable to record specific events, including the turning on and off of the monitor. Some monitors can record continuously, and most can be interfaced with a pulse oximeter to record drops in oxygen saturation that can occur with apneic events.

The information that is recorded by the memory monitor can be downloaded into a computer. This information is analyzed and quantified, with a resultant printout of use times, actual events, and event logs; ECG; oxygen saturation; and other data. The physician can use this information to make clinical decisions, including whether to continue or discontinue monitoring. Some physicians request documented monitoring as a routine part of cardiorespiratory monitoring of their patients. Funding by third-party payers for documented monitoring is not universal, and it is important to establish coverage before placing this type of monitor on an infant.

More extensive monitoring is also undertaken in the home using multichannel physiologic studies. These studies allow for the identification of central, obstructive, and mixed apneic events as well as ECG, nasal airflow, oxygen saturation, and diaphragmatic movement. Esophageal pH and breath hydrogen testing can also be performed with these multichannel recording devices to test for esophageal reflux.

Follow-Up for the Monitored Baby

Monitoring can be a stressful event for parents and families; because of this, extensive teaching and counseling may be required for some families. The home care RCP is responsible for educating the family in the appropriate use of the monitor and will then use subsequent visits to assess the family and provide reinstruction as indicated. The home care RCP should review any event logs kept by the parents and may collect them to send to the physician. The home care RCP should also verify the presence of extra supplies such as electrodes and lead wires. At least one extra set of monitoring supplies should be on hand at all times. The parents should be encouraged to ask questions or provide any observations they may have.

Frequency of home visits should be based on the clinical needs of the infant and family. Monthly visits may be necessary to download the memory from a recording monitor. The HME provider should have an RCP available on a 24-hour basis to address problems that develop after business hours. Maintaining close contact with the family and providing ongoing support will help make monitoring less stressful.

The Pediatric Tracheostomy

The Tracheostomy Tube

A major difference in the pediatric tracheostomy patient is in the tracheostomy tube itself. These tubes are much smaller and shorter, with inner diameters ranging from 2 to 7 mm. Neonatal, infant, and pediatric tracheostomy tubes do not have a cuff. It is believed that the narrow lumen created by the cricoid cartilage acts as a "cuff" for the tracheostomy tube. Pediatric and adult tracheostomy tubes are made of the same materials: silicone and polyvinyl chloride.

The smaller inner diameter of the pediatric tube increases the possibility of occlusion with secretions. Pediatric tracheostomy tubes are too small to have an inner cannula (the inner cannula in the adult tube can be removed and cleaned frequently, reducing the chance of occlusion). For this reason, every person caring for the child with a tracheostomy tube must be trained to change it in an emergency situation.

Changing the Tracheostomy Tube

Adult tracheostomy tubes are generally changed monthly or even less frequently if cuffless. Pediatric tracheostomy tubes are changed much more frequently, sometimes as often as once a week or more to help reduce the risk of occlusion.[19]

A real problem with tracheostomy tubes occurs as the child becomes older. Older children often try to decannulate themselves. This is another reason for every person caring for the pediatric tracheostomy patient to be trained in the rapid replacement of the tracheostomy tube. The risk of accidental decannulation can be reduced by making sure the tracheostomy ties are kept snug by tying the twill in a square knot. Velcro tracheostomy tube holders are also useful in reducing the risk of accidental decannulation.

Another factor to consider is the need to replace the tracheostomy tube as the child grows. Failure to change to a larger tube as the child becomes older will increase the airway resistance of the tube, particularly when the child is being mechanically ventilated.

Suctioning

Endotracheal suctioning of the pediatric patient is performed using essentially the same technique as that used for adults, whether mechanically ventilated or spontaneously breathing.[20] Children commonly need suctioning at bedtime, upon awakening, and before naptime.[19] Home suction machine pressure should be regulated to be as low as possible to remove secretions.[20]

Suctioning the pediatric tracheostomy patient is commonly accomplished in one of two ways. Most secretions can be cleared from the tracheostomy tube with the use of a shortened suction catheter. A pediatric suction catheter is trimmed to approximate the length of the tracheostomy tube. The use of this modified catheter greatly reduces the irritation and trauma to the trachea and carina that can occur with suctioning. A common nasal bulb syringe is also used to remove secretions that are visible at the hub of the tracheostomy tube.

Deep suctioning is performed using conventional suction technique. Instillation of a few drops of normal saline is recommended only for removal of thick secretions and should not be a routine part of the suction procedure.[21,22] Suctioning is typically performed using either a modified sterile (nonsterile gloves, sterile suction catheter) or clean technique (nonsterile or no gloves, clean suction catheter). Suction catheters are routinely rinsed through with boiled or distilled water, dried by suctioning air through them, and saved for reuse.

Vocalization

A very important aspect of the growth of a child is the development of speech. Infants use their voices to communicate their needs through crying. They make and repeat sounds to achieve coordination of oral structures associated with speech. The infant who has a tracheostomy cannot communicate by crying or making other sounds. These children often suffer developmental delays because of the tracheostomy.[23] It is essential to evaluate the child with a tracheostomy for communication. Several methods can be used to enhance the ability of these children to communicate. These include speaking valves and tracheostomy tube plugging.

The use of a simple one-way valve attached to the tracheostomy (Fig. 4–5) has enabled many children (and adults, for that matter) to communicate through vocalization. The valve opens during inspiration and closes during exhalation, forcing the exhaled air up through the vocal cords and out through the nose and mouth.

The decision to use a speaking valve should be made by the physician and the speech pathologist while the child is still in the hospital. The child must be evaluated and monitored during the initial trial phase to ensure tolerance. The physician will write orders for specific times that the valve should be used as part of the discharge plan.

The home care RCP must understand the use of the speaking valve to train other caregivers. The caregivers must be trained in attaching the valve to the tracheostomy tube and in identifying difficulties the child may experience with the valve. They must also clean the valve according to the manufactur-

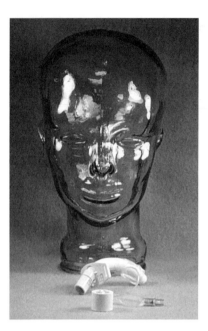

FIGURE 4–5
One type of speaking valve used on the pediatric patient.

er's specifications. The RCP will work in conjunction with the speech therapist to ensure continued success with using the valve as the child grows.

Children requiring mechanical ventilation at night or who are tracheostomized and do not require mechanical ventilation may tolerate having their tracheostomy tube "plugged" or capped during the day. The child should be carefully monitored for respiratory distress during plugging. Some children are also taught to plug the tracheostomy tube with their finger during speech.

Humidification

Many adults with tracheostomy tubes go through life without externally humidified air. The increased risk of occlusion by secretions and the potential for hypothermia caused by inhaling cold air require that pediatric tracheostomy patients have their inspired air heated and humidified. This is accomplished with the use of heated humidifiers and heat and moisture exchangers, commonly known as hygroscopic condenser humidifiers (HCHs) or "artificial noses."

Heated humidifiers may be included in-line as part of the ventilator circuit or used for continuous aerosol to the tracheostomy. The heating device should be servo-controlled, and the temperature should be monitored at all times to keep the inspired gas at 33°C $\pm$ 2°.[24] Infants and small children are more prone to hypothermia and hyperthermia, necessitating the continu-

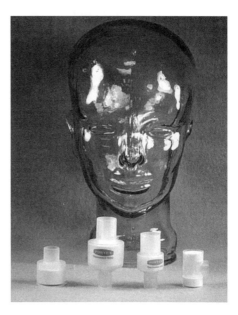

FIGURE 4–6
Artificial noses of different sizes.

ous monitoring of inspired air temperature. Wick- and passover-heated humidifiers are most commonly used in the home.

It is difficult to take along a humidifier or aerosol-generating device when the child is taken outside the home, and it may be cumbersome to set up this equipment when the child is taken off the ventilator for weaning trials or free time. The pediatric tracheostomy patient who is not on a ventilator also needs humidification. HCHs are very useful in these circumstances. These devices retain heat and moisture from the child's exhaled air, which is then used to warm and humidify the child's next breath.

Criteria for use of the artificial nose in the pediatric patient are the same as in an adult: It should not be used for the patient with copious secretions that repeatedly obstruct the device. The child should be capable of tolerating the resistance to inspiration that the HCH may cause. The RCP must be aware of the different sizes of artificial noses to choose the most appropriate size for the child (Fig. 4–6). Great caution must be taken when using an artificial nose on a ventilator-dependent child, as the low-pressure alarm on the ventilator may be ineffective because of the resistance of the HCH.[24]

Home Ventilator Care

Discharging a child who requires continuous ventilatory support is occurring with greater frequency. Children from every age group who may have previously spent their entire lives in the hospital are now being sent home.

Being part of the team making possible the discharge of a pediatric ventilator patient is a very rewarding experience.

The process of discharging any ventilator patient is complex and beyond the scope of this book. The reader is urged to consult the numerous texts available that deal specifically with this subject. Refer also to the bibliography on mechanical ventilation in Chapter 3.

Other Equipment

At times, the home care RCP sets up other types of equipment that are considered nursing-related because most HME companies do not employ both a nurse and an RCP. There are many times when the home care RCP will deliver the equipment and provide the initial instruction, and then the patient is followed by the home health nurse. The home care RCP must receive special training before setting up equipment that is not respiratory therapy–related.

Phototherapy

Phototherapy lights are a type of equipment not traditionally set up by RCPs in the hospital but are commonly set up by home care RCPs. Phototherapy lights are used to treat hyperbilirubinemia in newborns. Bilirubin is processed in the liver, where it is broken down to components that are excreted by the bowel. Some newborns have livers that are slow to function, causing the bilirubin to build up in the bloodstream. This buildup causes the newborn's skin and conjunctiva to take on a yellowish hue known as jaundice.

In previous times, babies were kept in the hospital to receive treatment for hyperbilirubinemia. They were forced to lie for hours at a time, unclothed and with eye covers to protect their eyes, in special beds that housed special overhead lights. Mothers either were kept in the hospital with these babies or were sent home without them. Phototherapy treatment could last for several days until the liver began processing the bilirubin on its own.

Technology has changed the treatment of hyperbilirubinemia dramatically. These babies can now be treated at home with "blanket"-type panels infused with fiber-optic lights (Fig. 4–7). The panel is wrapped around the baby's thorax, and the baby can then be wrapped in a blanket. Keeping the baby in a blanket eliminates the need for eyepatches. Using the fiber-optic panel rather than overhead lights also allows the parents to hold their baby, promoting the bonding that is essential during the baby's first few days of life.

The home care RCP will set up and instruct the parents in the use of the phototherapy lights. The physician will indicate the number of hours per day that the baby should be using the lights, as well as the intensity of the light in some instances. Treatment may last from 1 or 2 days to several days, depending on the baby's liver function. Follow-up for this type of patient will include

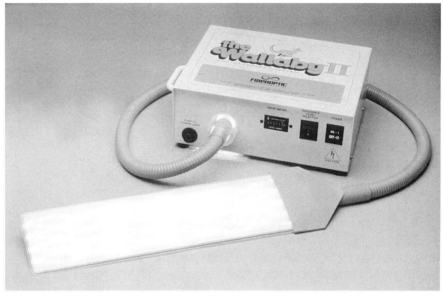

FIGURE 4–7
Blanket-type phototherapy lights.

evaluation of use times and any problems the parents may have encountered, as well as the amount of disposable supplies remaining.

Babies who are treated at home with phototherapy require daily blood draws for bilirubin levels. A nurse from a home health agency will come to the home to draw the blood sample, or the parents may be asked to take the baby to a laboratory. As the liver becomes able to process bilirubin, the blood level of bilirubin drops.

Feeding Pumps

The RCP may be requested to set up an enteral therapy pump, more commonly known as a feeding pump, for a pediatric patient. A feeding pump is a fairly simple device that carefully regulates the amount of liquid nutrition delivered to a feeding tube that has been inserted in the stomach or jejunum of an infant or child who is unable to take food by mouth. Feeding pumps are either electric- or battery-powered; some come in small carrying pouches that hold both the pump and the bag of liquid food, called a pumpset. These portable pumps are ideal for the older child who goes to school (Fig. 4–8).

The home care RCP generally instructs the family and other caregivers in setting the flow rate on the feeding pump, as well as teaches them to fill and attach the pumpset and maintain the battery. The home care RCP will also teach the family and other caregivers to troubleshoot problems with

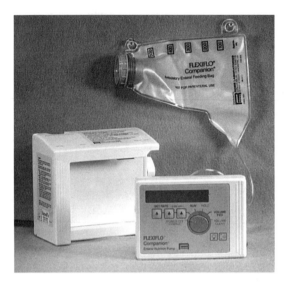

FIGURE 4–8
Portable feeding pump.

the pump or pumpset but will not instruct them in problems occurring with the feeding tube. Most pediatric patients with a feeding pump are also being followed by home health nurses, who will assist the family in maintaining the feeding tube.

SUMMARY

The major barrier to pediatric home respiratory care today continues to be cost and coverage. While the cost savings as compared with hospital stay are significant, it is substantial for the family when out-of-pocket expenses are incurred. Legislative attempts to seek provision of funding for health care are ongoing, but the system remains inadequate for today's increasing needs. Insurance companies often have a cap on a particular coverage, which may not be adequate for long-term needs, not to mention rising costs for premiums and yearly deductibles. The future of successful home care will be determined by its affordability with regard to adequate coverage, and the issue will repeatedly be addressed as a major topic in health care provision. Nevertheless, capable families with the advantages of funding, detailed planning, training, and appropriate outside support can benefit from caring for their child at home and can significantly enhance the quality of life for both family and child.

The RCP who provides pediatric respiratory home care feels the satisfaction of assisting in the discharge of a child after many months in the hospital. Helping that child by providing the equipment that allows the child to go to school and participate in other activities that are normal for children can be one of the most rewarding experiences the home care RCP can have. The RCP who understands the challenges and differences of pediatric respiratory home care is a valuable member of the home health care team.

REFERENCES

1. Merritt, TA, Northway, WA and Boynton, BR: Contemporary Issues in Fetal and Neonatal Medicine: Bronchopulmonary Dysplasia. Blackwell Scientific Publications, Philadelphia, 1986, p 3.
2. Lee, KS et al: Neonatal mortality: An analysis of recent improvement in the United States. Am J Public Health 70:15–21, 1980.
3. DeWitt, PK: Obstacles to discharge of ventilator-assisted children from the hospital to home. Chest 103:1560, 1993.
4. Make, BJ et al: Mechanical ventilation beyond the critical care unit: Report of a consensus conference of the American College of Chest Physicians. Chest Oct 1997, in press.
5. Goldberg, AI and Frownfelter, D: The ventilator-assisted individuals study. Chest 98:428–433, 1990.
6. Deming, DD: Respiratory assessment of neonatal and pediatric patients. In Wilkins, RL, Krider, SJ and Sheldon, RL (eds): Clinical Assessment in Respiratory Care, ed 3. Mosby-Year Book, St Louis, 1995, p 195.
7. Larter, NL and Miller-Ratcliffe, M: Special considerations for children. In Turner, J, McDonald, G and Larter, N (eds): Handbook of Adult and Pediatric Respiratory Home Care. Mosby-Year Book, St Louis, 1994, p 50.
8. Groothius, JR and Rosenberg, AA: Home oxygen promotes weight gain in infants with bronchopulmonary dysplasia. American Journal of Diseases in Children 141:992, 1987.
9. Thomas, RB et al: Psychosocial care of families and children. In Turner, J, McDonald, G and Larter, N (eds): Handbook of Adult and Pediatric Respiratory Home Care. Mosby-Year Book, St Louis, 1994, p 319.
10. Venkataraman, ST et al: Pediatric respiratory care. In Dantzker, DR, MacIntyre, NR and Bakow, ED (eds): Comprehensive Respiratory Care. WB Saunders, Philadelphia, 1995, p 1004.
11. Perinatal-Pediatric Focus Group: AARC clinical practice guideline: Selection of an aerosol delivery device for neonatal and pediatric patients. Respiratory Care 40:1325, 1995.
12. Meliones, JN et al: Pathophysiology-based approach to neonatal respiratory care. In Dantzker, DR, MacIntyre, NR and Bakow, ED (eds): Comprehensive Respiratory Care. WB Saunders, Philadelphia, p 1033.
13. Perinatal-Pediatric Focus Group: AARC clinical practice guideline: Selection of an oxygen delivery device for neonatal and pediatric patients. Respiratory Care 41:637, 1996.
14. Groothius, JR, Louch, GK and Van Eman, C: Outpatient management of the preterm infant. Respiratory Therapy 9:69, 1996.
15. National Institutes of Health: Consensus Statement of Infantile Apnea and Home Monitoring. Bethesda, MD, US Department of Health and Human Services, Public Health Service, Oct 1986.
16. Sheldon, SH, Speire, JP and Levy, HB: Pediatric Sleep Medicine: Sleep-Disordered Respiration in Childhood. WB Saunders, Philadelphia, 1992.
17. Spitzer, AR and Fox, WW: Infant apnea. Pediatr Clin North Am 33:561, 1986.
18. Hunt, CE: SIDS update: What we know—what we still don't know. Respiratory Therapy 9:79, 1996.

19. Mizumori, NA et al: Mechanical ventilation in the home. In Turner, J, McDonald, G and Larter, N (eds): Handbook of Adult and Pediatric Respiratory Home Care. Mosby-Year Book, St Louis, 1994, p 273.
20. Mechanical Ventilation Guidelines Committee: AARC clinical practice guideline: Endotracheal suctioning of mechanically ventilated adults and children with artificial airways. Respiratory Care 38:500, 1993.
21. Ackerman, MH: The effect of saline lavage prior to suctioning. Am J Crit Care 2:326, 1993.
22. Hagler, DA and Traver, GA: Endotracheal saline and suction catheters: Sources of lower airway contamination. Am J Crit Care 3:444, 1994.
23. Albamonte, S et al: Pediatrics. In Mason, MF (ed): Speech Pathology for Tracheostomized and Ventilator Dependent Patients. Voicing!, Newport Beach, CA, 1993, p 383.
24. Mechanical Ventilation Guidelines Committee: AARC clinical practice guideline: Humidification during mechanical ventilation. Respiratory Care 37:887, 1992.

chapter 5

Infection Control

Susan L. McInturff, RCP, RRT
Patrick J. Dunne, MEd, RRT

Protecting the Patient
Who Is at Risk
Common Sites of Infection
Community-Acquired Pneumonia
Transmission of Pathogens
Prevention

Protecting the Caregiver
Occupational Hazards
Human Immunodeficiency Virus
  and the Respiratory Care
  Practitioner

Identifying Risks
Immunizations
Appropriate Precautions

Equipment Cleaning and Disinfection
The Cleaning Procedure
Educating Patients and Caregivers
Surveillance

Summary

Infection control is of great concern for the home care RCP, but it is also very inexact. A wealth of information is available regarding infection control in the acute care setting; the Centers for Disease Control and Prevention (CDC), in particular, has established guidelines specific to hospital infection control practices. Nurses also have guidelines regarding infection control in acute and home care settings. Even the respiratory care community has established recommendations for infection control as it pertains to the use of equipment in the hospital. There are no unique guidelines, however, for infection control specific to the home care RCP.

The CDC defines a health care worker as "any person, including students or trainees, whose activities involve contact with patients or with blood or other body fluids from patients in a health care setting."[1] This definition then includes the home care RCP as well as family members and any other caregivers in the home. Although guidelines have been established by the CDC and other organizations specifically for infection control in the hospital, these guidelines are useful to home health care providers. The home care RCP can use these guidelines not only in practice but also in teaching the patient and caregivers about infection control procedures they will be performing.

This chapter outlines aspects of infection control that are essential knowledge for the home care RCP. The types of patients at risk for infection are identified as well as means of pathogen transmission to these patients. The primary focus is on protecting the patient, but emphasis is also placed on protecting the RCP and the patient's caregivers. Common methods of cleaning and disinfecting home respiratory equipment are also presented.

Protecting the Patient

The primary goal of any health care worker is to protect patients and "above all else, do no harm." One way to protect the patient is to reduce the patient's risk of infection. The home care RCP should make every attempt to reduce any possibility of transmitting infectious microorganisms to the patient or from an infected patient to others.

The RCP working in the acute care setting is familiar with the term "nosocomial infection." A nosocomial infection is one that is acquired while a patient is in the hospital and that is neither present nor incubating on admission.[2] This term does not apply to infections acquired outside the acute care setting; rather, these infections are considered "community-acquired." Many infections that occur in the home care setting are acquired in the same manner as those that are considered nosocomial, such as through direct contact or through certain care procedures. Although these infections cannot be strictly defined as nosocomial, the home care RCP must use similar infection control precautions to ensure that the patient does not become infected in this way.

Who Is at Risk

The home care RCP assists in the treatment of individuals who are at exceptional risk for infection. Many of these patients have one or more medical conditions that put them at substantial risk. Table 5–1 outlines medical conditions commonly seen in the home care setting that put patients at risk for infectious complications.

As Table 5–1 illustrates, virtually all patients who are followed by the home care RCP are at some degree of risk. It has been estimated that home care patients have an average of 3.6 comorbid medical conditions and are immunosuppressed relative to other people in the community.[3] The existence of comorbid conditions increases a patient's risk for infection. It is important

TABLE 5–1
**FACTORS THAT PUT A PATIENT AT
INCREASED RISK FOR INFECTION**

- Extremes in age (less than 5 years, greater than 65 years)
- Primary diagnosis of chronic obstructive pulmonary disease (COPD), cardiac disease, diabetes, cancer, or stroke
- Immunosuppression
- Tracheostomy
- Mechanical ventilation
- Presence of a urinary drainage catheter
- Presence of an intravenous catheter
- Presence of a nasogastric tube
- Comorbid conditions such as COPD, cardiac disease, diabetes, cancer, and stroke

to bear this in mind, particularly when the RCP may be informed only of the patient's primary diagnosis.

The RCP can use the initial patient interview to identify risk factors. Questions should be asked of the patient and family to identify the history of the patient's primary illness and any other diagnoses. The RCP should also establish any past medical history, familial medical history, and any environmental factors that could put the patient at increased risk of infection. Types of environmental factors that the RCP should look for are poor housekeeping or sanitation, source of water (well or city), and types of cleaning facilities available.

The patient interview will also assist in identifying the patient who was treated for an infection while in a health care facility and determining whether that infection is still being treated. The home care RCP should review the patient's discharge orders, medication schedule, and home nursing care plan. This review can help identify any indicators for potential infections, such as orders for antibiotics or antifungal agents, orders for cultures, or change in wound status.[4]

Common Sites of Infection

It is important for the home care RCP to understand which patients are at an increased risk of infection. It is also important for the RCP to understand which sites of the body are most prone to infection. The most common sites for infection seen in home care are the urinary tract, wounds, and lower respiratory tract.[3]

Urinary tract infection is the most common type of infection seen in the home.[4] Patients requiring an indwelling bladder catheter or intermittent bladder catheterization or patients whose bladders do not empty completely during urination are at the greatest risk.

Open wounds also present a special risk to the home care patient. Certain medical conditions and medications can cause the skin to tear easily with only the slightest bump. Elderly patients can often be seen with such wounds. Moreover, these wounds may not heal very rapidly. Other types of wounds are tracheostomy and transtracheal stoma. These conditions must be recognized and treated as open wounds, even if they are well healed. Any break in the skin, whether surgical or accidental, increases the patient's chance of infection.

The home care RCP may not play a role in the identification or treatment of urinary tract or wound infections (except for tracheostomal infections) but should be aware of their presence. Sequelae from these infections, such as fever, pain, and discomfort, can have an impact on the patient's breathing, requiring assessment and possible intervention and treatment. More importantly, the home care RCP should be aware that these types of infections are present so that the RCP does not spread infectious pathogens to other sites on the patient's body or to any other patient.

Community-Acquired Pneumonia

Another type of infection common to the home care patient is pneumonia. Overall, pneumonia is the sixth leading cause of death in the United States, and it ranks as the number one cause of infection-related death.[5] Patients on assisted mechanical ventilation via tracheostomy have the highest risk of contracting pneumonia.[6]

Pneumonia contracted outside the acute care setting is considered to be community-acquired.[5] Because community-acquired pneumonia is so prevalent and so life-threatening, home care RCPs must have a clear understanding of the means of protecting the patient from pneumonia-causing pathogens. Common microorganisms attributed to community-acquired pneumonia in elderly patients with comorbid conditions are[5]:

- *Streptococcus pneumoniae*
- *Haemophilus influenzae*
- Respiratory viruses
- *Legionella*
- *Mycobacterium tuberculosis*

It is important to remember that most home care patients with pneumonia do not have a sputum culture performed to identify the infectious organism. Instead, physicians usually treat patients with broad-spectrum antibiotics that are effective against the most common pneumonia-causing organisms. Because of this practice, the home care RCP may never know which organism caused the pneumonia and, therefore, should focus on preventing the transmission of all infection-causing microbes.

TABLE 5–2
MEDICAL CONDITIONS THAT PROMOTE COLONIZATION (PER THE CENTERS FOR DISEASE CONTROL)

- Alcoholism
- Diabetes mellitus
- Pulmonary disease
- Coma
- Hypotension
- Acidosis
- Conditions that require a nasogastric tube
- Conditions that require an endotracheal tube/tracheostomy
- Conditions that require the use of antimicrobials
- Malnutrition

Transmission of Pathogens

Many patients receiving home care have been discharged from the hospital colonized with low levels of the very microbes that can infect them later. Disease states commonly seen in the home care patient tend to promote colonization of pathogens in the oropharynx, tracheobronchial tree, and stomach.[6] Table 5–2 lists several of these common diseases.

Once the patient is colonized, the infectious pathogen can invade the lower respiratory tract, bladder, or wounds in several ways. Table 5–3 reviews these routes of transmission.

Aspiration

A problem very common to home care patients is aspiration. The presence of a tracheostomy tube, dysphagia, or gastric reflux can greatly increase the risk for and complications of aspiration. Invasion of the lower respiratory tract with colonized oropharyngeal or gastric secretions will inevitably lead to infection.

TABLE 5–3
ROUTES OF TRANSMISSION FOR COLONIZED MICROBES

- Via aspiration of oropharyngeal and gastric flora
- Via the "conduit" provided by an endotracheal tube
- Via inhalation of droplet nuclei
- Via hands (cross-contamination)
- Via contaminated respiratory care equipment

The RCP should be on the alert for patients who are prone to aspiration and assist in protecting the lower airway. Keeping the head of the bed elevated during sleep can help, as will proper inflation of the tracheostomy tube cuff, if one is in place. An evaluation by a speech pathologist is extremely helpful in identifying problems with swallowing and dysphagia. Withholding food for several hours before bedtime and controlling the flow of enteral feeding via a nasogastric tube can help reduce the potential for aspiration. A feeding tube implanted in the stomach or jejunum may be indicated for patients with serious aspiration and dysphagia problems.

Endotracheal Intubation

A patient with an endotracheal tube is at an increased risk for infection because the tube acts as a conduit to the lower airway, not only for air but for bacteria as well. Infectious microorganisms can be introduced into the lower airway by way of a suction catheter as it is passed through the endotracheal tube, and contaminated oropharyngeal secretions can leak past an inflated cuff on the tracheostomy tube.[6] It has been shown that patients on continuous mechanical ventilation are up to 21 times more susceptible to the development of nosocomial pneumonia.[6] We might infer from this statistic that home ventilator patients are also more susceptible and that infection control procedures should be practiced accordingly.

Droplet Transmission

Pneumonia can also be caused by the inhalation of microorganisms that are transported via droplets generated during sneezing, coughing, and talking. Contaminated droplets can also be generated during suctioning. These droplets are propelled only a short distance and are deposited onto the receiver's nasal mucosa, mouth, and conjunctivae. Common infectious microbes that are transmitted in this manner are *Haemophilus influenzae*, the togavirus that causes rubella, adenovirus, the influenza virus, and *Streptococcus*.

Airborne Transmission

Infection-causing microorganisms can also be transported by droplet nuclei or dust particles. Droplet nuclei are "small-particle residue (5 μg or smaller in size) of evaporated droplets containing microorganisms that remain suspended in the air for long periods of time."[7] The microorganisms can be inhaled by a susceptible patient who is in the *same room* as an infected person. *Mycobacterium tuberculosis* and *Varicellavirus* are examples of infectious microorganisms that are spread by inhalation.

Cross-Contamination via Hands

One of the first things RCPs learn when beginning their work in the hospital is to *wash their hands,* and for good reason. Contact transmission is the most frequent mode of transmission of nosocomial infections,[8] and we must assume that this is true for home care as well. Cross-contamination occurs when contaminated hands are not washed or gloves are not changed after patient contact. It also occurs when hands are not washed or gloves are not changed before moving from one part of the body to another between procedures.

Patients receiving home care will frequently have many different people touching them, including themselves. The RCP will touch the patients when shaking hands; auscultating breath sounds; evaluating ankle edema; and during suctioning, tracheostomy care, and other procedures. The home health nurse will touch patients in similar ways, perform wound or bladder care, or assist patients with bathing or their bowel program. Family members may come in close contact by kissing or hugging the patient, and they may also perform many of the procedures usually done by the RCP and the nurse. The patient may also be responsible for cross-contamination; consider the tracheostomy patient who uses the bathroom and then uses his or her finger to occlude the tracheostomy tube to speak.

Contaminated Respiratory Therapy Equipment

Many of the devices used in respiratory care come in contact with the patient's mucous membranes and respiratory tract. These devices are frequently filled with water or a water-based liquid to produce aerosols. Nosocomial infections have often been attributed to using contaminated respiratory therapy equipment.

Home respiratory therapy devices that have been contaminated can also pose risks to home care patients. Home oxygen equipment may be set up with bubble humidifiers, many patients use medication nebulizers, and even home ventilators and continuous positive airway pressure (CPAP) machines use passover or heated humidifiers.

The key problem with home respiratory therapy equipment is that it is not subjected to the type of disinfection that is carried out in the hospital. Most home respiratory therapy equipment is cleaned by the patient. Home care patients do not use autoclaves or gas sterilizers, and glutaraldehyde solutions are not commonly used in the home.

Prevention

The RCP with an understanding of at-risk populations and pathogen transmission is armed with the information needed to minimize the patient's exposure. The primary method of prevention is through isolation precautions.

The RCP in the hospital is accustomed to using isolation precautions for infection control. The patient's hospital room may have a sign on the door identifying necessary isolation procedures and barriers, such as gloves, gown, goggles, or mask. The patient's chart will also identify which types of infection control procedures are necessary and, especially, why. Home care RCPs may not have such information available to them, however.

Standard Precautions

Remembering that virtually all home care patients are at greater risk for infectious complications, the home care RCP must use *standard precautions and transmission-based isolation procedures* for *all* patients.[8] These precautions were developed by the CDC specifically for hospitals, but the lack of guidelines specific to home respiratory care justifies the modification and implementation of hospital guidelines to the home care setting.

Standard precautions and transmission-based isolation procedures combine the major features of the former universal precautions and body substance isolation. Standard precautions apply to "(1) blood, (2) all body fluids, secretions, and excretions *except sweat,* regardless of whether they contain visible blood, (3) nonintact skin, and (4) mucous membranes."[8] Standard precautions call for handwashing before moving from one body site to another during procedures, handwashing between patients, and handwashing after removing gloves, even if another pair of gloves will be put on. An easy rule to remember is this: If your hands could get wet, wear gloves.[9] *Wearing gloves is not a substitute for handwashing in any instance.* Depending on the circumstances, additional barrier protective devices (gowns, goggles, face shields) may also be necessary. Table 5–4 outlines standard precautions and transmission-based isolation procedures.

The home care RCP must be prepared for any level of isolation precautions that may be called for by having an infection control kit available at all times. Table 5–5 lists the items that should be included in the kit. It should be carried in the home care RCP's vehicle and restocked whenever anything is taken from it.

Immunizations

Immunization is one of the most important ways of preventing infection. A patient who is elderly and has chronic cardiopulmonary disease can suffer grave consequences if he or she contracts such common diseases as influenza or pneumonia. Most adults have been either immunized or exposed to

TABLE 5–4
**STANDARD PRECAUTIONS AND TRANSMISSION-BASED
ISOLATION PROCEDURES TO BE USED ON *ALL* PATIENTS**

A. Handwashing with antimicrobial soap
  ● After touching body fluids, secretions, blood, contaminated items
  ● After removing gloves
  ● Between procedures on different body parts
B. Gloves
  ● Wear when touching blood, body fluids, etc.
  ● Change gloves between tasks
C. Mask, eye protection, face shield
  ● Wear to protect mucous membranes when performing procedures
    that are likely to generate splashes or sprays
D. Gown
  ● Use to protect skin and clothing during procedures that generate
    splashes or sprays

communicable diseases such as measles, diphtheria, and varicella. Many, however, do not become immunized against influenza and pneumonia.

The CDC recommends that an annual influenza vaccine be given to any person at high risk for developing infectious complications.[10] Table 5–1 identifies these high-risk patients. Annual vaccination is necessary because of the continuous mutation of the influenza virus. People remain susceptible to the influenza virus all their lives because, although they develop antibodies to the virus, those antibodies do not protect them from the mutated virus. The vaccine should be administered to high-risk patients from mid-October to mid-November each year.

The CDC also recommends that people who are considered high risk receive the pneumococcal vaccine. *Streptococcus pneumoniae,* or pneumococ-

TABLE 5–5
**THE INFECTION CONTROL KIT
TO BE CARRIED IN THE HOME
CARE RESPIRATORY CARE
PRACTITIONER'S VEHICLE**

Kit should contain:

● Nonsterile gloves
● Masks
● Goggles or other protective eyewear
● Disposable gowns
● Infectious and noninfectious waste containers
  (red and clear plastic bags)
● Antiseptic no-rinse hand cleaner
● Alcohol wipes
● Spray disinfectant

cus, is considered to be the pathogen most often associated with community-acquired pneumonia.[5]

The current pneumococcal vaccine is polyvalent and will immunize against 23 strains of pneumococcal bacteria. This vaccine was preceded by a 14-valent vaccine, which was replaced by the current vaccine in 1983. The pneumococcal vaccine needs to be given only once. People previously immunized with the 14-valent vaccine should be reimmunized with the 23-valent vaccine.

The RCP can use the patient interview to establish whether the patient has received these immunizations. Nonimmunized patients should be strongly advised to contact their physicians.

Protecting the Caregiver

As important as it is to ensure that the patient is protected from infection, it is also very important for home care RCPs to protect themselves from contracting infections from the patient. The patient's caregivers must also learn this aspect of infection control.

Occupational Hazards

Clinicians in the acute care setting are very aware of the hazards and risks of caring for patients with communicable diseases. They understand that the hospital is an environment teeming with infectious agents. Fortunately, policies, procedures, and guidelines abound to help the hospital-based RCP. Hospitals have isolation rooms, signs, goggles, masks, gowns, and other methods to alert and protect the staff.

The home care RCP must understand that there are also serious risks outside the hospital. A principal hazard is that a patient's infectious condition may be not be known to the home care RCP. One reason for this situation is that the referral source may be trying to protect the patient's right to privacy and may not identify the infectious condition when calling to order home medical equipment. It is not unusual for the home care company to be called to set up a piece of equipment for an adult patient whose diagnosis is suspect for an underlying infectious condition. For example, a referral source might give a patient's diagnosis as cytomegalovirus (CMV). This diagnosis might cause the RCP to speculate whether this patient has acquired immunodeficiency syndrome (AIDS) because CMV is fairly uncommon in adults except when the patient is immunocompromised. The potential for a patient to have an underlying infectious condition is very real.

The home care RCP must also be mindful of "silent" infections such as methicillin-resistant *Staphylococcus aureus* (MRSA), hepatitis B, and human immunodeficiency virus (HIV). The patient may have received treatment for these conditions in the hospital so that the conditions are not considered a hazard to caregivers outside the hospital. Patients who have been treated for such infections may continue to be colonized, however, and could cross-contaminate themselves, the home care RCP, and other caregivers during close contact.

Another common risk is that of treating the child who has respiratory syncytial virus (RSV). For example, the home care RCP may be called on to set up a compressor-nebulizer for a child who has just been diagnosed with the virus and is leaving the emergency room. Patients with RSV secrete large numbers of the virus via droplet nuclei, and the virus is known to survive on inanimate objects for hours. The RCP could easily contaminate his or her hands with the virus during the nebulizer setup and then transfer the virus to his or her nasal mucosa or conjunctivae without even being aware of its happening.[6] These children are frequently discharged from the emergency room or doctor's office with their parents' receiving little instruction on preventing the spread of RSV. This practice is significant, considering that children who are hospitalized with RSV are placed in some type of isolation. In fact, the CDC now recommends that patients with RSV remain isolated until their course of treatment is completed.[8] Because home care patients, including children, are seldom placed in isolation, the home care RCP must use extra caution when working with these patients.

Human Immunodeficiency Virus and the Respiratory Care Practitioner

Transmission of HIV in the home care setting is considered to be rare.[11] The virus is not easily transmitted by skin or mucous membrane exposure to HIV-infected blood. The risk of transmission is even less for exposure to secretions without visible blood.[11] Studies show that few, if any, RCPs have acquired HIV infections through exposure while on the job.[12]

Percutaneous exposure to HIV by needlestick presents a greater risk than skin or mucous membrane exposure; however, the home care RCP does not use a needle percutaneously on a patient very often. Some home care RCPs perform arterial punctures, but this service is provided by very few home care companies. Syringes with needles are used more often for drawing up medications such as gentamicin or pentamidine for use in medication nebulizers.

Although the occupational risk of contracting HIV is very, very low, the potential for exposure certainly exists. The greatest danger to home care RCPs is that they will not know that the patient is HIV-infected. Exposure can occur while the RCP performs such common procedures as suctioning or bagging the patient and collecting a sputum sample. With proper precautions, these procedures can remain low risk.

TABLE 5–6
**IMMUNIZATIONS RECOMMENDED BY
THE CENTERS FOR DISEASE CONTROL
FOR ALL HEALTH CARE WORKERS**

- Hepatitis A
- Hepatitis B
- Influenza
- Measles
- Mumps
- Rubella
- Pneumococcus
- Tetanus
- Varicella (with no history of chicken pox and
  with negative blood titer)

Identifying Risks

The best way for the home care RCP to reduce the risk of contracting an infection or becoming contaminated is to continually *be aware.* To assume that a patient does not pose any risk just because he or she is not in the hospital is naive and potentially dangerous thinking.

The patient interview is the most important tool in assisting the home care RCP to identify any conditions that pose an infectious risk. For example, during the compressor-nebulizer setup for the child whose diagnosis is given as "acute bronchiolitis," the RCP may discover that the child tested positive for RSV. Asking the parent or caregiver which antibiotics the child was placed on or what types of medical tests were ordered can provide useful information.

There are times, however, when the home care RCP may not be able to obtain the information needed to identify an infectious risk. The patient or caregivers may be unable to remember what medical tests were performed or why. They may be uncomfortable or reluctant to answer the RCP's questions about medications or other health issues. In these types of situations, the home care RCP might consider contacting the patient's physician to inquire about suspected infectious conditions if there are any concerns.

Immunizations

It is recommended that *all* health care workers be immunized against several common communicable diseases. Table 5–6 lists these immunizations.[13] Some home medical and respiratory therapy equipment (HME/RT) companies request proof that a prospective home care RCP has been immunized as a condition of employment.

Appropriate Precautions

Because most home care patients are at risk for infection and the home care RCP may not be aware of the presence of an infectious condition, it is essential to take appropriate precautions. The home care RCP must *always assume* that there is a risk for contamination or infection.

Given this assumption, home care RCPs must have the means to protect themselves. This is accomplished primarily by practicing the same standard precautions that are used to protect the patient. Nonsterile gloves must be worn any time the RCP will come in contact with blood or body fluids, secretions, or excretions. This could occur during such procedures as suctioning, demonstrating tracheostomy care or tracheostomy tube insertion, or setting up a nebulizer for a baby who is coughing or drooling. Gloves are not necessary when performing procedures such as chest auscultation, blood pressure reading, or other procedures on dry, intact skin. Hands *must* be washed after removing gloves and after touching the patient. The importance of handwashing by *all* members of the respiratory home care team (patient, family members, caregivers, and RCP) cannot be overemphasized.

There may be times when just donning gloves does not offer enough protection, for example, during suctioning of a patient whose diagnosis is suspicious for an underlying infection. The infection control kit that is carried in the vehicle should have available all the barriers necessary to provide ample protection for the visiting RCP.

Equipment Cleaning and Disinfection

Just as there are no universal guidelines for infection control in home care, there are also no universal guidelines for the cleaning and disinfection of home care equipment. The consensus seems to be that home care equipment *should* be cleaned, but there is little agreement on frequency of cleaning. There are also disparate opinions about disinfection versus sterilization and whether home care equipment must undergo this level of processing at all (and, if so, how often).

It is important to understand the meaning of the terms that are used in conjunction with this aspect of infection control. "Cleaning" is the process by which any foreign material (dirt, dust, secretions, medications, etc.) is removed from an object. "Disinfection" is the process that removes pathogenic microorganisms from an inanimate object. "Sterilization" is the process that destroys all forms of microbial life.[14]

Disinfection and sterilization procedures are also categorized as high level and low level. *High-level* disinfection and sterilization procedures are carried out by subjecting the equipment to wet heat pasteurization at 76°C for 30 min. These procedures are also carried out by using liquid chemical disinfectants/sterilants that have been approved as such by the Environmental Protection Agency. An HME/RT company subjects equipment to high-level disinfection and sterilization between patients. *Low-level* disinfection is accomplished using solutions such as acetic acid (vinegar) or quaternary ammonium compounds. Low-level disinfection is the method used most frequently by home care patients.

The Cleaning Procedure

There is no standard method for cleaning and disinfection of home respiratory equipment. The American Respiratory Care Foundation (ARCF) published recommendations in 1988, and, although these may be the only guidelines directed specifically to home respiratory care equipment,[14] they may not reflect prevailing practices. A majority of equipment manufacturers have specific cleaning and disinfection procedures that they recommend for their equipment, but, of course, these guidelines vary among manufacturers.

The key to equipment maintenance and infection control is education and training. If patients and caregivers understand why it is so important to clean and disinfect their equipment, they may be more likely to comply. Making the process as simple as possible and providing step-by-step written instruction will markedly improve compliance.

Hospitals and HME/RT companies have dedicated areas for clean and dirty equipment. The home care patient, however, may not have a separate area of the home solely for this purpose. Kitchens and bathrooms are frequently used, but these rooms, of course, are used for other purposes as well.

Because patients may have no special *area* to use for cleaning equipment, it is helpful for them to have a *container* solely for this purpose. Kitchen and bathroom sinks can harbor soap and oil residues as well as bacteria that might adhere to the surfaces of the equipment; using a designated container will eliminate this problem. The container (bowl, bucket, or other appropriately sized container) can be placed in the sink during cleaning and then stored when not in use. The bathroom is not an acceptable place for cleaning equipment because of the infectious microorganisms that may be present in the spray created during flushing of the toilet.

Home medical equipment should be cleaned regularly, although there is no consensus on frequency. Some HME companies and manufacturers recommend daily cleaning and disinfection, while others recommend cleaning less frequently and may feel that disinfecting the equipment is unnecessary. Patients and caregivers often make their own decisions about how frequently (or infrequently) they will clean their equipment, particularly if they are trying to save money on disinfectant solutions or if the procedure is too complex for them.

TABLE 5-7
SAMPLE CLEANING/DISINFECTION PROCEDURE

- Wash hands.
- Set up cleaning area, supplies.
- Disassemble equipment.
- Wash parts in hot, soapy water using antimicrobial dish detergent in container designated for this purpose. Use a brush to clean parts as necessary.
- Rinse parts thoroughly with tap water to remove all traces of soap.
- Place parts on paper towel to dry, or
- Prepare disinfectant solution according to manufacturer's instructions, or
- Mix 1 part white vinegar to 3 parts tap water.
- Completely submerge parts in disinfectant or vinegar solution. Be sure that the insides of tubings and parts are completely covered by the disinfectant or vinegar solution. Soak in disinfectant for manufacturer's specified length of time or soak in vinegar solution for 30 min.
- Rinse parts thoroughly in tap water.
- Place parts on paper towel to dry.
- When parts are completely dry, wash hands in antimicrobial soap and reassemble parts. Place them in a paper bag until ready for use.
- Keep disinfectant covered between uses, and use only as long as recommended by the manufacturer. Vinegar solution should be discarded after each use.

Table 5-7 outlines a sample cleaning/disinfection procedure. This procedure is based on prevailing practice but does not include frequency. The ARCF recommendations that were published in 1988 recommended *daily* cleaning and disinfection of home medical equipment. The CDC has more recently recommended that respiratory care equipment such as ventilator circuits and humidifiers *not* be routinely changed more frequently than every 48 hours.[6]

Even though the CDC guidelines were written to direct hospital infection control practices, it is reasonable to expect that home respiratory care equipment would not require changing more frequently than every 48 hours. Most patients and caregivers can easily remember an "every other day" schedule, or a "Monday-Wednesday-Friday" schedule.

Educating Patients and Caregivers

As essential as it is for the home care RCP to understand infection control, it is equally important for the patient and caregivers to understand this process. A significant way to protect the patient from infection is through adequate education and training. The patient and caregivers must realize the reasons for infection control, means of infectious organism transmission, and methods of avoiding infection transmission to the patient.

Most hospitals have an infection control specialist whose function is to provide educational programs and ongoing training in infection control procedures to the hospital staff. Studies show improvement in staff compliance with infection control procedures following in-service education for

TABLE 5–8
SIGNS AND SYMPTOMS OF INFECTION

- Localized redness, swelling
- Fever, generalized malaise
- Pain at site
- Abnormal drainage at site
- Increased cough
- Increased sputum production
- Color change in sputum (yellow, green)

these procedures.[13] This knowledge can be applied to the home care setting: Patients and caregivers who receive ongoing education and training will be more compliant with the procedures they are being asked to perform.

Training must begin very early on and may need to be repeated several times to ensure that the patient and caregivers understand the infection control procedures and can adequately perform them. It is ideal to train the patient and caregivers while the patient is still in the hospital. If hospital training was not provided, infection control training must begin during the RCP's first home visit. The training should include proper handwashing technique and practical demonstrations of equipment disassembly and cleaning/disinfection. Patients and caregivers should also be taught to recognize common signs and symptoms of infection (Table 5–8).

Patients and caregivers should also be educated in the proper handling and disposal of potentially hazardous materials. If a patient is using a suction machine, the contents of the suction canister should be emptied into the toilet, not into the kitchen or bathroom sink, where it could potentially come in contact with skin or mucous membranes. The suction canister itself should be cleaned and disinfected.

Solutions remaining in humidifiers or other water reservoirs should be emptied into the sink or toilet and replaced daily, and the humidifier or water reservoir should be cleaned and disinfected with the same frequency as the rest of the patient's equipment. Prefilled humidifiers or other prefilled water reservoirs should be discarded and replaced when they have reached their minimum fill level.

Surveillance

During home visits, the RCP should evaluate the patient and caregivers for their ability to perform infection control procedures as instructed. Their compliance with these procedures should also be evaluated. Such evaluations can be made by observing the patient and caregivers as they perform procedures such as suctioning and tracheostomy care, equipment cleaning, or even administration of a nebulizer treatment. The home care RCP can observe the patient and care providers to determine whether handwashing takes place before and after performing care procedures.

The care providers can be questioned about their method of preparing disinfectant solutions, how often the solutions should be changed, and how the equipment is stored after cleaning. It may also be helpful to observe the equipment cleaning and disinfection process as it is performed. Any deviation from the originally taught procedure must be evaluated to determine whether it is acceptable, and any unacceptable procedures must be retaught.

SUMMARY

The ultimate goal of the home care RCP is to transfer responsibility for the care of patients afflicted with chronic medical conditions to the patients themselves. This goal is particularly important when it comes to infection control. Patients, family members, and other caregivers must "buy in" to the concept that they are responsible for reducing the risks of infection for the patient. The home care RCP can assist patients and their families in assuming these responsibilities through education and training.

Home care RCPs must emphasize handwashing, provide clear and easy-to-follow instructions for equipment cleaning and disinfection, and teach patients ways to reduce the risk of infection. Armed with this information, patients should then be capable of managing their own infection control.

Home care RCPs must also reduce the risk of carrying infectious organisms to other patients. Before this can happen, however, the home care RCP must have a clear understanding of infection transmission, at-risk individuals, and methods of prevention. Although no specific guidelines currently exist for infection control in respiratory home care, *general* guidelines can be applied to the home care setting. These guidelines will help home care RCPs protect the patients, the caregivers, and themselves.

REFERENCES

1. Clever, LH and LeGuyader, Y: Infectious risks for health care workers. Annu Rev Public Health 16:141, 1995.
2. Bergogne-Berezin, E: Treatment and prevention of nosocomial pneumonia. Chest 108:26s, 1995.
3. Smith, PW: Infection prevention in the home health setting. Asepsis 16:9, 1994.
4. Rosenheimer, L: Establishing a surveillance system for infections acquired in home healthcare. Home Healthcare Nurse 3:20, 1995.
5. Mandell, LA: Community-acquired pneumonia. Chest 108:35s, 1995.
6. Hospital Infection Control Practices Advisory Committee, Centers for Disease Control

and Prevention: Guideline for prevention of nosocomial pneumonia. Respiratory Care 12:1191, 1994.

7. American Thoracic Society: Control of tuberculosis in the United States. Respiratory Care 8:929, 1993.

8. Hospital Infection Control Practices Advisory Committee, Centers for Disease Control and Prevention: Guideline for isolation precautions in hospitals, Part II. Recommendations for isolation precautions in hospitals. Am J Infect Control 1:32, 1996.

9. Valenti, WM: Infection control, human immunodeficiency virus, and home health care: II. Risk to the caregiver. Am J Infect Control 23:78, 1995.

10. Centers for Disease Control and Prevention: Influenza and Influenza Vaccine: The Flu. Information Pamphlet. US Department of Health and Human Services, Public Health Service, Bethesda, MD, March 1995.

11. Centers for Disease Control and Prevention. Human immunodeficiency virus transmission in household settings—United States. JAMA 24:1897, 22/29 1994.

12. Luce, JM: HIV, AIDS, and the respiratory care practitioner. Respiratory Care 2:189, 1993.

13. Diekema, DJ and Doebelling, BN: Employee health and infection control. Infect Control Hosp Epidemiol 16:292, 1995.

14. American Respiratory Care Foundation. Guidelines for disinfection of respiratory care equipment used in the home. Respiratory Care 9:801, 1988.

chapter 6

Reimbursement

Lia Shaw Miller, BA, RCP
Patrick J. Dunne, MEd, RRT

The RCP receives comprehensive training to perform many aspects of respiratory care. This training prepares the RCP to make sound decisions and deliver appropriate care. However, one aspect of respiratory care for which RCPs receive little or no training is reimbursement. The lack of training in this very important area poorly prepares the RCP for the realities of health care today.

Most RCPs enter the work force without much concern for the way in which the procedures they perform are paid for and by whom they are paid. The RCP may be aware that Medicare exists but may know little more than the fact that retired people have Medicare. The RCP may work in a hospital owned by a managed care organization but may not understand managed care's effect on the patient's medical care.

The acute care RCP may administer oxygen to a patient without ever having to consider whether that patient's insurance will pay for it. Disposable supplies are used freely without the RCP's having to consider whether the patient's insurance has limits on those supplies. The RCP may believe that the patient needs an oximeter to monitor oxygen saturation upon discharge to home and may be surprised to find that the patient's insurance company believes an oximeter is not medically necessary. The fact is that RCPs can no longer assume that just because they believe something is necessary or because the physician prescribes it, the insurance company is going to pay for it. RCPs cannot even assume that *their* services are going to be paid for.

This chapter provides the RCP with an overview of the mechanics of reimbursement. The major types of health insurance programs are described, and coverage guidelines for home respiratory care are outlined. Armed with this information, the RCP will better understand reimbursement issues' effects on health care in general and on respiratory care in particular.

The Basis of Health Care Reimbursement

The financing of health care services in the United States originates from three basic sources: (1) federal and state governmental programs (i.e., Medicare and Medicaid), (2) private insurance programs, and (3) private pay. Medicare and Medicaid evolved in response to the problem of unaffordable health care for certain groups of the population (i.e., Medicare for the elderly and Medicaid for the economically disadvantaged). Once implemented, however, health insurance programs such as Medicare and Medicaid were major contributors to a nationwide increase in the demand for and availability of health care services.

Some economists see the availability of health insurance as a driving force in the rapid escalation of the cost of health care. Financial obstacles to attaining health care were minimized with the introduction of health insurance. The notion that "someone else" was paying the bill encouraged both providers and consumers to take full advantage of growing technological advances. Further, the mechanism developed to reimburse hospitals, physicians, and other health care providers contributed, in large part, to health care inflation. Hence, we are now witnessing in this country major changes in the way all health care services are being reimbursed. The concept of "managed care" plays a principal role in the radical change in the way in which health care is financed in both the private and public sectors.

Since 1965, providers of home respiratory therapy equipment services have labored under reimbursement policies that are now viewed as archaic and shortsighted. It is hoped that health care restructuring will result in rational and defensible reimbursement mechanisms for these providers, because the demand for such services is not expected to abate anytime in the foreseeable future.

TABLE 6–1
MEDICARE AS IT IS ADMINISTERED BY THE DEPARTMENT OF HEALTH AND HUMAN SERVICES

Health Care Financing Administration (HCFA)	Social Security Administration (SSA)
Defines Medicare benefits	Processes Medicare applications
Sets Medicare rates	Determines eligibility
Administers Medicare program	Issues Medicare card
Contracts for claims payment	Provides public information

Medicare

The Medicare program is a federal health insurance program that was signed into law in 1965 by President Lyndon Johnson as Title XVIII of the Social Security Act. Initially, Medicare was intended to provide health insurance for the elderly, those aged 65 years or older. The program was expanded in 1972 to also cover people under age 65 who were medically disabled as well as those with end-stage renal disease (ESRD). Medicare is administered through fiscal intermediaries (Part A) and regional carriers (Part B) under the direction of the Health Care Financing Administration (HCFA). HCFA is a division of the Department of Health and Human Services (DHHS). Table 6–1 traces Medicare as it is administered by DHHS.

There are two separate, distinct benefits within the Medicare program: (1) Medicare Part A, Hospital Insurance, and (2) Medicare Part B, Medical Insurance. Medicare Part A covers in-patient acute hospital services, care in a skilled nursing facility, intermittent home health care visits, and hospice care. Medicare Part A has deductibles and co-insurance, but the majority of beneficiaries do not have to pay premiums for Part A.

Medicare Part B covers physician services, outpatient therapy and hospital services, durable medical equipment (DME), and ambulance services. For most services covered under Part B, the beneficiary is required to pay an annual deductible ($100 in 1997) and co-insurance, typically 20 percent of the amount allowed by Medicare. A more complete description of coverage under Medicare Part A and Part B is seen in Table 6–2.

Payroll taxes finance the Medicare Part A Hospital Insurance trust fund. Payroll taxes also finance the Old Age and Survivors Disability Insurance (OASDI) trust fund. Fully 132.9 million workers paid Federal Insurance Contributions Act (FICA) or Self-Employment Contributions Act (SECA) taxes on wages earned during 1992. An inspection of a payroll stub identifies these taxes that are taken out to finance Medicare Part A Hospital Insurance. Medicare Part B, a *voluntary* supplementary medical insurance program, is funded through a combination of monthly premiums paid by beneficiaries (25 percent) and general revenues (75 percent). The

TABLE 6–2
MEDICARE PART A AND PART B COVERED SERVICES

Medicare Part A (1997 deductible: $760)	Medicare Part B (1997 premium: $43.80; annual deductible: $100)
Hospitalization: Semiprivate room and board, general nursing, and other hospital services and supplies	Medical expenses: Doctors' services, inpatient and outpatient medical and surgical services and supplies, physical and speech therapy, diagnostic tests, durable medical equipment and other services
Skilled nursing facility care: Semiprivate room and board, skilled nursing and rehabilitative services and supplies	Clinical laboratory services: Blood tests, urinalyses, and more
Home health care: Part-time or intermittent skilled care, home health aide services, durable medical equipment and supplies, and other services	Home health care: Part-time or intermittent skilled care, home health aide services, durable medical equipment and supplies, and other services
Hospice care: Pain relief, symptom management, and support services for the terminally ill	Outpatient hospital treatment: Services for the diagnosis or treatment of illnesses or injury
Blood: When furnished by a hospital or skilled nursing facility during a covered stay	Blood

Medicare Part B monthly premiums are typically withheld from the beneficiary's Social Security check.

In 1994, a total of almost 36 million beneficiaries, composed of 32 million elderly and 4 million disabled persons, were covered by Medicare. Enrollment for the elderly has grown an average of 2 percent per year since the program's inception. Enrollment of the disabled has grown an average of 3.9 percent per year since the program was expanded in 1972. A relatively small number of beneficiaries qualify because they have ESRD.[1] Not every beneficiary who is covered under Part A Hospital Insurance is also covered under Part B (because it *is* voluntary), a fact that can be very problematic for providers of home medical equipment.

Enrollment in Medicare can be automatic or voluntary. The importance of this distinction is that it determines whether a person is entitled to receive Part A benefits without paying a monthly premium (ranging from $187 to $311 in 1997, depending on the number of quarters paid into Social Security). Persons are automatically eligible for Medicare if they are:

- Eligible for Social Security Administration Title II Retirement
- Eligible for Civil Service and Railroad Retirement
- Social Security and Railroad Retirement Disability recipients (disabled for 24 full months)
- Diagnosed with end-stage renal disease (ESRD)
- Persons who turned age 65 before 1975 but do not qualify for Social Security benefits ("traditional" eligibility)

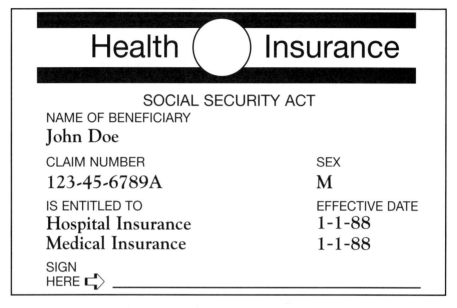

FIGURE 6–1
Example of a Medicare card.

Persons who turned age 65 between 1968 and 1975 can receive Medicare if they have a certain number of "covered quarters of work," even though they may fall short of qualifying for Social Security. Local Social Security offices can determine eligibility.[2]

Medicare beneficiaries are issued a red, white, and blue Medicare card that identifies their health insurance claim (HIC) number. This Medicare number is usually the beneficiary's Social Security number or that of their spouse. The Medicare card also lists beneficiary's coverage. Figure 6–1 is an example of a Medicare card; the home care RCP may be asked to view a patient's Medicare card to verify whether the patient has both Medicare Part A and Part B. Because Part B is the coverage that reimburses for DME, the lack of it can pose a problem. The patient without Part B coverage is required to pay for the medical equipment themselves; however, many patients will not want the equipment if they have to pay for it out of their own pocket.

Medicare and Managed Care

Medicare beneficiary enrollment in managed care programs is a relatively new phenomenon but is already growing at an annual rate of 31.2 percent. As of March 1997, more than 5 million Medicare beneficiaries have enrolled in some form of managed care organization (MCO). Recent HCFA studies project that, given the current uncertainty surrounding health care reform and the pending insolvency of the Medicare Trust Fund, by the year 2000 almost 50 percent of Medicare beneficiaries will be covered by a managed care health plan.[3] To date, the growth of Medicare enrollment in managed care plans has been concentrated in a few large states such as California, New York, and Florida. This picture is expected to change rapidly as health maintenance organizations (HMOs) and other managed care plans broaden their reach and influence.

Medicare and the Home Medical Equipment Industry

The home medical equipment (HME) provider that supplies equipment for a Medicare Part B beneficiary can bill Medicare directly for that equipment. The provider can "accept assignment" for the equipment, meaning the provider accepts the allowable dollar amount that Medicare pays for that equipment and Medicare will then send the money directly to the provider. For example, the HME company may provide an oxygen concentrator to a patient and agree to accept assignment. The company will bill Medicare for the retail rental price of the concentrator, $325 per month. However, because the company accepts assignment, it agrees to accept the $300 per month that Medicare allows for a concentrator. Medicare will send the company *80 percent* of $300, and then the patient is responsible for the remaining *20 percent* (recall that the patient is required to pay the co-insurance, typically 20 percent of the amount allowed by Medicare). The difference between the retail rental price of $325 and the Medicare allowable amount of $300 is "written off" by the company as a contractual allowance.

If a company *does not* accept assignment, the patient is charged the entire retail price, and the company may bill Medicare as a service to the patient. Any payment made by Medicare is sent directly *to the patient;* this payment is 80 percent of Medicare's allowed charge, not the company's retail charge. Using the example of the concentrator again, the patient is charged $325 and the company sends a complimentary billing to Medicare for $325. Medicare sends the patient 80 percent of its allowed charge of $300. The remaining $25 is considered an out-of-pocket expense of the patient.

Most DME companies agree to accept assignment and bill Medicare for services that are a benefit of the Medicare program. However, if a service is not a benefit of Medicare, the company is not likely to accept assignment. For example, the company will probably agree to accept assignment for a compressor-nebulizer, but it will not accept assignment on a grab bar for the patient's bathroom. Medicare pays for compressor-nebulizers but does not pay for bathroom safety aids.

Although most home care RCPs are not involved in billing Medicare, they will frequently hear the phrase "accept assignment" and are often asked questions about Medicare by the patients they see. A good working knowledge of what Medicare is, who has it, and how it works is extremely helpful to the day-to-day practice of the home care RCP.

Medicaid

Medicaid, a jointly funded federal and state medical assistance program for the economically disadvantaged, was enacted in July 1965 through Title XIX of the Social Security Act. The program was designed to provide health insurance coverage to persons with limited assets based on means testing. Medicaid is funded by matching federal and state contributions, and, although some rules are established by federal law, its specific financial eligibility and outline of coverage are largely determined and regulated at the state level. Forty-nine states, the District of Columbia, Puerto Rico, the Virgin Islands, Guam, American Samoa, and the Northern Mariana Islands all operate Medicaid programs. Arizona operates a federal assistance program as an alternative to Medicaid under a waiver of some basic federal requirements.

Medicaid serves primarily three groups of people: (1) low-income mothers and children who use acute and ambulatory services similar to those covered by private health insurance, (2) nonelderly disabled persons who use both health insurance services and long-term care, and (3) low-income elderly persons who use Medicaid to supplement their Medicare benefits; e.g., Medicaid will pay the deductibles and co-insurance the patient is normally responsible for.

In 1993 Medicaid spending was about $125 billion. Children represent half of all beneficiaries, but they incur the lowest cost per person. The highest spending is for disabled adults and the elderly. This is partly due to the fact that Medicaid is one of the largest funders of long-term care, paying 53 percent of all nursing home care.[4] Services that are generally offered through the Medicaid program include the following:

- Physician's services
- Inpatient and outpatient hospital services
- Skilled, intermediate, and custodial nursing facility care
- Home health care
- Family planning services
- Rural health clinic services

The individual states have some range in defining the benefits and eligibility criteria for Medicaid in their respective jurisdictions. For institutional care under the Medicaid program, an individual must have certification from a physician that a specific level of care is necessary, for example, skilled, intermediate, or custodial care. This certification must be renewed by the physician every 6 months.

Medicaid also plays a role in home- and community-based care through the Medicaid Waiver programs. Medicaid Waiver programs allow states greater flexibility in using Medicaid funds to provide these services as an alternative to institutionalized care. Medicaid Waiver programs are commonly used to fund the care of ventilator- and other technology-dependent children and adults at home

Many states "contract" with a single HME provider for respiratory services. This means that, if a patient needs a respiratory service like oxygen, only the contracted provider can supply it to the patient. This is important to know, particularly if the patient goes to a noncontracted provider to get the equipment. For example, the home care RCP on call for the weekend may receive a referral to supply a patient with a compressor-nebulizer. Upon delivery of the equipment, the RCP discovers that the patient has Medicaid, which is not a problem if the RCP works for the contracted provider. However, if the RCP works for a noncontracted provider, Medicaid is not going to pay that company for the compressor-nebulizer.

It is illegal for the company to bill the patient for the nebulizer once it learns that the patient has Medicaid. What usually happens is that the contracted provider is notified and it supplies the patient with a compressor-nebulizer. The noncontracted provider then retrieves its equipment. The home care RCP who is familiar with reimbursement issues and Medicaid will be able to determine whether the service is reimbursable *before* the service is provided.

Medicaid will often pay for items that are not covered by other payers, such as Medicare. This can work to the patient's advantage, particularly when the patient requires supplies for tracheostomy or other ostomy care, incontinence, or bathroom safety aids. Specialized wheelchairs or other seating devices are also frequently covered by Medicaid upon evidence of medical necessity. Coverage varies from state to state, and the home care RCP would be well served to become familiar with what is and what is not covered by Medicaid in his or her state.

Private Commercial Insurance

Private insurance is a nongovernmental source for the financing of medical services. Historically, health insurance was instituted as a method of redistributing the financial risk associated with major illnesses from individuals to collectives mediated by insurance companies. Insurance was developed to protect people from economic losses. Health insurance companies function as the channel between individuals and their doctors, hospitals, and any other health care providers. They function by taking in a predetermined amount of money per person covered (the "premium") and paying it out as costs are incurred. Premiums are based on the insurance companies' best estimate of the average cost to cover enrolled individuals for a defined set of health benefits.

There are two types of private health insurance: "group" plans and "individual" plans. A group insurance plan is one in which an insurer issues a "master" insurance policy to an employer, association, or other entity to provide benefits for its members or employees. The employee or member in turn receives a "certificate of insurance" that summarizes the provisions of the master insurance policy. Changes can occur in benefits or premiums, or the policy can be canceled as a result of a third party, the "group" holding the master policy.[5] Group insurance is most commonly offered as a benefit of employment or membership in an association.

An individual insurance policy is a written contract between an insurance company and an insured person. In general, to purchase this type of plan a person must provide evidence of insurability to the insurance company through detailed health questionnaires. An insurer has the right to decline coverage on the basis of the applicant's personal habits (for example, alcohol or nicotine addiction), medical history, age, income, or any number of other factors. Generally, the cost of individual health insurance coverage is higher than group plans because of the increased degree of risk.

Some private commercial insurance companies have agreements with health care providers to provide services to their beneficiaries. These agreements may or may not be exclusive. "Participating providers" agree to provide their services at a contracted rate that is generally lower than their retail rate. Patients who receive health care services from participating providers may not have to pay the co-insurance, typically 20 percent of the paid amount.

There is a wide variation in benefits and coverage among the different types of commercial insurance plans. Because of this variability, most HME providers try to verify coverage before providing a service to a client. This contact will verify whether the patient has coverage for the service in question as well as the amount of insurance coverage and the patient's co-insurance amount. This contact will also verify whether the insurance company has participating providers. Depending on the co-insurance amount or the participation of a preferred provider, the patient may not wish to have the service provided by the HME company.

Payment Methods

Two traditional methods are used by third-party payers to compensate providers of health care services: (1) prospective payment and (2) fee-for-service. Prospective payment plans pay a specific amount for a specified occurrence or an amount based on the actual diagnosis. Actual charges are not taken into account under prospective payment.

On the other hand, fee-for-service benefits are generally paid as a percentage of the approved charge for a "covered" service, such as 80 percent of the allowed charge of a doctor's office visit. Under traditional Medicare, most of Part A acute hospital benefits are paid prospectively using diagnosis-related groups (DRGs); HCFA has determined how much the hospital care should cost to treat a patient with a particular diagnosis and will pay the hospital that amount, regardless of the hospital's actual cost of care.

The majority of Medicare Part B benefits are paid under a fee-for-service schedule. HCFA has again determined the amount the fees should be for specific Part B services, known as the "allowed" charge. Most insurance companies pay under a similar fee-for-service schedule; in fact, many insurance companies follow Medicare's guidelines for payment.

Managed Care

The concept of managed care in the United States dates back to 1929. At that time in Elk City, Oklahoma, a physician named Michael Shadid established a rural farmers' health cooperative in a community of 6000 with no medical specialists, selling shares to raise money for a new hospital and establishing annual dues to cover the costs of care.[6] By 1934, 600 family memberships supported a medical staff that by then included Dr. Shadid, four new specialists, and a dentist who had relocated to the area. Another significant milestone in the evolution of managed care occurred in 1934, when two Los Angeles physicians, Drs. Donald Ross and Clifford Loos, entered into a prepaid contract to provide comprehensive health services to 2000 employees of a local water company.

Between 1930 and 1960 several other major prepaid group practice plans began, including the Group Health Association in Washington state in 1937, the Kaiser Permanente Medical Care Program in Northern California in 1942, and others. These organizations encountered strong opposition from organized medicine, but they also experienced significant success in attracting enrollees.[7]

Managed care has as its primary objective the control of health care expenditures through the rigorous management of the use of health care resources. Managed care is different from conventional health insurance in that a managed care organization either provides the services directly (e.g., Kaiser Permanente) or enters into contracts with other providers to obtain necessary services for its members. A conventional third-party insurer, in contrast, underwrites the care without ever becoming directly involved in the delivery system.

Managed care comes in three major forms: (1) managed fee-for-service with case management/utilization review oversight, (2) preferred provider organizations (PPOs), and (3) health maintenance organizations (HMOs). The managed fee-for-service type of reimbursement is a modified version of the traditional fee-for-services form but with the payer (HMO, PPO, or IPA) having the power to authorize or deny reimbursement for medical services. PPOs contract with a limited number of physicians and hospitals who agree to provide care for plan members, generally on a discounted fee-for-services basis. HMOs combine insurer and providers into one entity.

HMOs come in two major types. In the independent practice association (IPA) model, one or more HMOs contract with a network of private physicians and hospitals to provide the total health care for a defined number of members in a defined geographical area. The group-model or staff-model HMO brings physicians and hospitals together under one organizational umbrella.

HMOs typically pay physicians and hospitals by "capitation" or salary. Capitation payment (for example, a monthly per capita payment, or payment "by the head") can be complex. A two-tier payment structure exists when the HMO pays capitation fees directly to the individual physician or small group practice without the use of the independent practice association (IPA). The three-tier structure involves an intermediary administrative structure for processing the capitation payment.[8] Typically, physicians remain in their own private offices but join together into IPAs. The IPA becomes the middle tier. Capitation payments are a fixed amount paid at predetermined time intervals. Payments are made for each patient assigned to a provider whether or not services are provided; conversely, providers are not reimbursed for services that exceed the fixed amount.

Cost containment has become an ever-growing concern of those who pay for health care in the United States. Fee-for-service, which encourages the use of more services, is being replaced with newer, more innovative reimbursement mechanisms. Managed care is changing the way in which health care is financed by changing the incentives in the health care system. Pressure is being placed on health care providers in all care settings to limit the quantity and intensity of services rendered to that which can be justified in terms of the member's medical condition and available resources. For some, managed care represents a dangerous threat to the nation's highly respected health care delivery system. What was once a source of revenue under fee-for-service becomes a cost under managed care. The argument against managed care is that physicians and other health care providers can make a profit only by providing less care. The argument against fee-for-service is that the provider profits when people are sick and use health services. Thus, there is less incentive to keep people healthy.

Theoretically, managed care can succeed by lowering costs for individual services and improving the efficiency of services provided to treat a specific illness. This can be accomplished by providing more effective care early, which may avoid higher-cost subsequent care. Additionally, by the substitution of less costly modes of care (e.g., outpatient versus inpatient surgery or transitional/nursing home or home care in place of acute hospital care), it may achieve the same ends less expensively.

Payment for Home Respiratory Therapy Equipment

Payment for home respiratory therapy equipment services is based on either rental or purchase of the particular item of equipment.[9] The standard rental period is 1 month. Coverage for the rental or purchase is predicated on medical necessity's being established by the prescribing physician.

Once medical necessity is established, the individual needing the equipment must have an insurance plan that includes an HME benefit. Medicare Part B is the most widely known benefit for home medical and respiratory therapy equipment. The second most popular source for this benefit is private commercial insurance plans. Historically, Medicaid plans vary widely from state to state with respect to coverage for home medical and respiratory therapy equipment services.

Documenting Medical Necessity

In addition to having medical necessity established by the prescribing physician and evidenced by the presence of a primary chronic pulmonary disease, most insurance payers for home respiratory therapy equipment also require supporting laboratory documentation to uphold the physician's prescription. For example, Medicare requires evidence of the presence of arterial hypoxemia, as supported by a resting room air arterial oxygen tension of 55 mm Hg or less, or the alternative, an arterial oxygen saturation of 88 percent or less. If the arterial oxygen tension is 56 to 59 mm Hg or the arterial oxygen saturation is 89 percent, a secondary diagnosis indicating the presence of cardiovascular deterioration as a result of the chronic hypoxemia is likewise required before coverage can be approved. Table 6–3 reviews Medicare's current coverage guidelines for home oxygen therapy equipment.

Home oxygen therapy equipment is presumed not to be medically necessary and will not be reimbursed for individuals with arterial oxygen tensions of 60 mm Hg or greater or arterial oxygen saturation at or above 90 percent, even if the prescribing physician feels that a regimen of home oxygen therapy is justified treatment. In these situations, alternative funding sources must be identified or private pay arrangements made.

Another example of additional laboratory documentation's being required to support reimbursement for home respiratory equipment is with nasal continuous positive airway pressure (CPAP) for treatment of obstructive sleep apnea. Evidence of obstructive sleep apnea must be provided in the form of a sleep study documenting at least 30 episodes of apnea, each

TABLE 6–3
CRITERIA FOR MEDICARE COVERAGE FOR HOME OXYGEN THERAPY

Oxygen therapy is covered for patients when there is:

- An arterial PO_2 at or below 55 mm Hg or an oxygen saturation at or below 88% taken at rest
- An arterial PO_2 of 56–59 mm Hg or an oxygen saturation of 89% with any of the following conditions:
  1. Dependent edema suggesting congestive heart failure;
  2. Pulmonary hypertension or cor pulmonale, determined by measurement of pulmonary artery pressure, gated blood pool scan, echocardiogram, "P" pulmonale of ECG (P wave greater than 3 mm in standard leads II, III, or aVF); or
  3. Erythrocythemia with a hematocrit greater than 56%
- An arterial PO_2 at or below 55 mm Hg or an oxygen saturation at or below 88% during exercise; in this case, oxygen will be covered during exercise if it is demonstrated that oxygen improves the hypoxemia that occurred while the patient was exercising on room air
- An arterial PO_2 at or below 55 mm Hg or an oxygen saturation at or below 88% taken during sleep; or a decrease in arterial PO_2 more than 10 mm Hg or a decrease in oxygen saturation more than 5% associated with signs or symptoms attributable to hypoxemia, such as nocturnal restlessness, insomnia, or impairment of cognitive processes; in these cases, oxygen will be covered for nocturnal use only

lasting a minimum of 10 sec during 6 to 7 hours of recorded sleep. Again, even if the prescribing physician feels that a patient has obstructive sleep apnea and that nasal CPAP therapy is indicated, Medicare will not reimburse for it without a qualifying sleep study.

Rental or Purchase

The decision to rent or purchase a particular piece of home respiratory therapy equipment rests solely with the third-party payer and is usually made on the basis of the proposed length of need and the complexity of the equipment being prescribed. For example, an insurance company may determine that it will not purchase a mechanical ventilator for a patient but will instead rent it. Because of the complexity of this particular piece of equipment, the type of maintenance it requires, and the type of patient that requires it, the insurance company may believe that the patient is better served by having the equipment rented. On the other hand, the insurance company may purchase a compressor-nebulizer at the outset, based on its relatively low cost and the likelihood of the patient's requiring its use in the future.

Current Medicare policy is to rent oxygen equipment, compressor-nebu-lizers, nasal CPAP and bilevel machines, mechanical ventilators, and suction machines. However, with the exception of oxygen equipment and mechani-cal ventilators, Medicare "caps" these rental payments after 15 months. This means that Medicare will pay the provider rent for the equipment for up to 15 months; after 15 months the patient can either purchase the equipment at his or her own expense or continue to use the equipment, and Medicare will pay the provider a maintenance fee once every 6 months. Oxygen equipment and mechanical ventilators are not capped rental items because they require frequent service to ensure continued optimum performance.

Monthly rental payments for home respiratory therapy equipment include the provision of all necessary accessories required for normal operation and function. This includes nasal cannulas, tubing, masks, headgear, humidifiers, and similar items. Accordingly, separate charges for replacement of such accessories and supplies are not covered. However, Medicare *does* provide additional reimbursement for certain supplies considered to be necessary for the normal operation of covered rental equipment. Examples are suction catheters, medications for compressor-nebulizers, and masks and accessories for CPAP.

Reimbursement for the Respiratory Care Practitioner in Home Care *there is none*

The delivery and setup of respiratory therapy equipment in the home presents a formidable challenge to HME providers. Evidence has repeatedly demonstrated that home respiratory therapy equipment is used best when a knowledgeable and experienced RCP is actively involved in the initial setup and training and is available to provide periodic follow-up visits to assess continued compliance and optimum equipment performance.[10] Regrettably, however, third-party payers, especially Medicare, do not recognize these professional home visits as being necessary and, accordingly, allow virtually no reimbursement for such visits. As cost-containment efforts intensify, it is unlikely that reimbursement rates for the rental or purchase of home respiratory therapy equipment will be raised in recognition of these added expenses. Rather, providers of home respiratory therapy equipment will be expected to continue to absorb the added costs of this valuable service with the hope that they will be able to offset to some degree the extra expense by continually improving the efficiency and effectiveness of their operational processes.

SUMMARY

The evolution of managed care came about in response to the rapidly increasing costs of providing health care services, and it is redefining the very fabric of health care delivery in this country. Providers (hospitals, doctors, and other suppliers of health care) are being scruti-nized by the payers of health care services, the government, and private insurance companies for every detail of the services they provide pertaining to medical necessity and cost efficiency. What used to take years to redesign is now changing in a matter of months in response to the demands of the system.

Managed care will continue to be a highly controversial yet visible part of the nation's health care delivery landscape at least through the end of the decade. Moreover, cost-containment pressures from both public and private sectors will fuel the growth of managed care for all age groups in all socioeconomic classes.

What does this portend for RCPs, especially those who have elected to pursue their career in home care? To maintain the competi-tive edge in this rapidly changing environment, the RCP must be informed, flexible, and ready to meet the challenges of managed care. In this area of cost shifting, the acute care setting is no longer the focal point of the health care environment, and the RCP will be more involved in home, community-based, and nursing home care. A major challenge posed by managed care will be the ongoing need to help those individuals working in a managed care organization in a deci-sion-making capacity to understand what home respiratory care ser-vices can contribute in terms of overall health care resource utiliza-tion.[11] Unfortunately, many well-intentioned case managers and utilization review practitioners simply lack experience with the HME industry in general and with home respiratory care in particular. Occasionally, they may not even be aware of what they do not know, and it will be up to experienced and knowledgeable RCPs to fill the often unappreciated role of educator.

REFERENCES

1. National Academy on Aging: Public Policy Report, Vol 7. National Academy on Aging, Portland, Maine, Nov 1995.
2. Health Care Financing Administration: 1996 Guide to Health Insurance for People with Medicare. US Department of Health and Human Services (Pub No HCFA-02110), Baltimore, Feb 1996.
3. Nevin, T: Medicare managed care enrollment grows at triple-digit rates in some states. Home Health Line 22:4–6,1997.
4. Medicaid Fact Sheet. Health Care Financing Administration, Baltimore, Nov 1995.
5. Department of Insurance: Consumers Guide to Group Health Insurance. State of California, Sacramento, 1988.
6. National LTC Resources Center: Managed Care Handbook for the Aging Network. Univer-sity of Minnesota, Minneapolis, Nov 1995.
7. MacLeod, GK: The Managed Care Handbook, ed 2. Aspen Publishers, Gaithersburg, MD, 1993.
8. Bodenheimer, T and Grumback, K: Reimbursing physicians and hospitals. Health care policy: A clinical approach. JAMA 272:971–977, 1994.

9. Dunne, PJ: Demographics and financial impact of home respiratory care. Respiratory Care 39:309, 1994.
10. Dunne, PJ: Using respiratory home care to reduce acute hospital utilization. The Case Manager 7:81, 1996.
11. National Association of Retail Druggists: Home Health Care Pharmacist 3:1, Alexandria, VA, October 1994.

■ *Glossary*

Activities of Daily Living (ADLs): Activities considered routine to everyday living, including walking, getting in and out of bed, bathing, dressing, eating, toileting, and taking medication.

Actual Charge: The amount a physician or other health care provider bills a patient for a particular medical service or procedure. This amount may differ from the Medicare-approved amount or the amount approved by other insurance programs.

Ambulatory Care: Health care services that are provided on an outpatient basis. No overnight stay in a hospital is required. Includes the services provided at ambulatory care centers, hospital outpatient departments, physicians' offices, and home health care services.

Approved Charge: The maximum fee that a third-party payer (insurer organization) will use in reimbursing a provider for a given service.

Assignment: The method of Medicare reimbursement in which a physician or supplier agrees to accept the amount approved by the Medicare carrier as total payment for covered services. The physician or supplier submits the claim on behalf of the beneficiary and is paid directly. In general, Medicare pays the physician or supplier 80 percent of the Medicare-approved amount, less the annual deductible. Beneficiaries are responsible for any part of the $100 annual deductible (1996) and the remaining 20 percent (co-pay) of the approved amount.

Beneficiary: Individual who either is using or is eligible to use insurance benefits, including health insurance benefits, under an insurance contract.

Capitation: A payment system in which managed care plans pay health care providers a fixed amount for providing services to a group of members over a given period. Providers are not reimbursed for services that exceed the fixed amount. The rate of reimbursement may be fixed for all members or it can be adjusted for the age and gender of the member, based on actuarial projections of medical utilization.

Certification of Medical Necessity (CMN): The statement by a physician regarding the medical necessity of a specific medical service or procedure.

Champus: The Civilian Health and Medical Program of the Uniformed Services is a government program that provides hospital and medical services to active duty and retired armed services personnel under age 65 and their eligible dependents.

COBRA: The Consolidated Budget Reconciliation Act of 1986 allows for workers who would otherwise lose their insurance coverage because of unemployment, divorce, or the death or retirement of a spouse to continue their group health insurance by paying their own premiums. The continuation policy is temporary and is available for 18, 19, or 36 months, depending on the reason for coverage. The law applies to private employers with 20 or more employees and to state and local government plans. Once COBRA coverage terminates, an individual is eligible to convert to an individual policy without qualifying based on preexisting conditions.

Coordination of Benefits (COB): Provisions and procedures used by insurers to avoid duplicate payment when an individual is covered by two or more health insurance plans. Coordination determines which insurer is the primary payer.

Co-payment: A specified dollar amount or percentage of health care costs that the beneficiary is required to pay.

Current Procedural Terminology (CPT): The listing of identifying codes for reporting medical services and procedures performed by physicians and other health care professionals.

Custodial Care: Care that is primarily for the purpose of meeting personal needs or activities of daily living and could be provided safely and reasonably by people without professional skills or training.

Deductible: A specified amount of medical expense that is initially due from the insured before payment will be made by the payer. Generally, deductibles must be met annually.

Diagnosis-Related Groups (DRGs): Payment categories used under Medicare's Prospective Payment System (PPS) in which Medicare reimburses hospitals a set rate for each DRG code.

Durable Medical Equipment (DME): To be considered durable medical equipment, the equipment must be able to withstand repeated use, serve primarily a medical purpose, and be appropriate for use in the home.

Durable Medical Equipment Regional Carrier (DMERC): A commercial health insurance company that contracts with the Health Care Financing Administration (HCFA) to process claims for Medicare Part B DME services.

End-Stage Renal Disease (ESRD): Medical condition in which a person's kidneys no longer function, requiring the individual to receive dialysis or a kidney transplant to sustain her or his life.

Explanation of Medicare Benefits (EOMB): The statement that informs beneficiaries and physicians about the action taken by the carrier in processing the Medicare claim. The notice includes information for both parties about their appeal rights and their liability for the cost of services.

Fee-for-Service: A payment system in which an amount is reimbursed for each encounter or service rendered. Payment is made after the fact.

Fiscal Intermediary: A private health insurance organization under contract with the Health Care Financing Administration (HCFA) to process Medicare Part A claims.

Gatekeeper: A primary care physician responsible for overseeing and coordinating all aspects of a patient's care under managed care plans.

Group Insurance: Any insurance policy or health services contract by which groups of employees (and dependents) are covered under a single policy or contract issued by the employer or other group entity.

Health Care Financing Administration (HCFA): The federal agency within the Department of Health and Human Services that administers the Medicare and Medicaid programs.

Health Care Financing Administration Common Procedure Coding System (HCPCS): HCPCS is a national uniform coding structure for reporting physician and supplier services under the Medicare program. HCPCS includes both the numeric procedure codes from the CPT and the alphanumeric codes and modifiers developed by HCFA and local Part B carriers.

Health Insurance Claim Number (HIC): The unique alphanumeric Medicare entitlement number appearing on the Medicare card assigned to a Medicare beneficiary.

Health Maintenance Organization (HMO): An organization that provides a comprehensive range of health benefits to an individual for a prepaid fee. An HMO contracts with health care providers, e.g., physicians, hospitals, and other health professionals, and members are required to use participating providers for all health services.

Indemnity: Traditional insurance programs that pay a fixed amount for covered services received. Generally referred to as Fee-for-Service programs.

Independent Practice Association (IPA): A health maintenance organization delivery model in which the managed care organization (MCO) contracts with a physician organization that, in turn, contracts with individual physicians. The physicians are members of the IPA, an independent legal entity, but maintain their own separate offices and identities. The HMO reimburses the IPA on a capitated basis.

International Classification of Diseases, 9th Edition, Clinical Modification (ICD-9-CM): Coding system of diagnoses required on all bills submitted for Medicare payment and most other third-party payers.

Medicaid: A joint federal-state health insurance program to finance health care services for low-income populations. It is financed by federal and state taxes.

Medicare: A federal health insurance program that provides coverage for persons over age 65, persons who have been disabled for 24 continuous months, and individuals with end-stage renal disease (ESRD). Part A of Medicare covers inpatient hospital services, skilled nursing care, home health care, and hospice; Part B of Medicare covers physician services, durable medical equipment (DME), clinical laboratory services, and other outpatient medical services.

Participating Physician: A physician who agrees in advance and in writing to accept assignment for all Medicare claims.

Preauthorization: A method of monitoring and controlling use by evaluating the need for medical service prior to its being performed.

Preferred Provider Organization (PPO): Organization in which insurers contract with a limited number of physicians and hospitals who agree to care for patients, generally on a discounted fee-for-service basis with utilization review. Beneficiaries have flexibility to use non-PPO providers, but usually at a higher cost.

Prospective Payment System (PPS): The standardized payment system implemented in 1983 by Medicare to help manage health care reimbursement, by which the incentive for hospitals to deliver unnecessary care is eliminated. Under PPS, hospitals are paid fixed amounts based on the principal diagnosis (DRG) for each Medicare hospital stay.

Reasonable and Necessary Care: The type and amount of health services generally accepted by the health community as being required for the treatment of a specific disease or illness.

Resource-Based Relative Value Scale (RBRVS): The RBRVS takes into account time, skill, and overhead expense in determining the value of a service. Multipliers or conversion factors are used with the total value units to determine the payment amount. Relative Value Scales are used by many PPOs and HMOs to set maximum allowable professional fees.

Secondary Payer: The payer of medical benefits after the primary carrier has paid its portion of the claim.

Share of Cost: For certain Medicaid beneficiaries, a specified dollar amount for medical services must be paid by the beneficiary each month before Medicaid benefits can be paid.

Third-Party Payer: The insurance company that pays hospital or physician bills for a beneficiary. Medicare supplemental insurance coverage is an example.

Utilization Review (UR): A systematic means for reviewing and evaluating the medical necessity, appropriateness, and quality of care.

chapter 7

Pulmonary Rehabilitation: Prevention, Not Just Treatment

Gerilynn L. Connors, RCP, RRT, BS, FAACVPR

Pulmonary rehabilitation (PR) has evolved over the years to become included as a standard medical therapy for pulmonary patients. The outcomes of PR are to control and alleviate symptoms and optimize functional capacity of the pulmonary patient. PR is a process that moves a patient toward better health and an increased level of wellness. PR is not only therapeutic but preventive as well.[1] PR should be considered for any patient with lung disease who is not able to function at his or her capacity. It is no longer acceptable to reserve PR for patients with end-stage lung disease and severe limitations of function. Patients must be referred to PR earlier in the course of their disease.[2]

The respiratory therapist and the PR specialist play vital roles in lung disease prevention by educating health care professionals and the general public about the importance of *early detection* of pulmonary disease through *screenings* such as *spirometry*. The simple spirogram should be considered for anyone with signs or symptoms of respiratory disease or with a smoking history. Macklem and Permutt in 1979 stated: "In considering the simplicity of determination of FEV_1 and its potential use in detecting individuals who are headed toward serious trouble at a time when intervention might have prevented a disastrous outcome, it is interesting to explore the reasons why the spirometer has not achieved a position comparable to the clinical thermometer, the sphygmomanometer, the ophthalmoscope, the chest x-ray and the EKG."[3]

The Definition of Pulmonary Rehabilitation

To have a historical understanding of PR it is helpful to know how rehabilitation has been defined over the years. In 1942 the Council of Rehabilitation defined rehabilitation as "the restoration of the individual to the fullest medical, mental, emotional, social, and vocational potential of which he or she is capable." PR addresses not only control of symptoms and disease but also health promotion and maintenance of health. Rehabilitation allows the patient to identify his or her "assets and liabilities," as well as the available choices for change.

In 1974, the American College of Chest Physicians adopted the following definition of pulmonary rehabilitation[4]:

> An art of medical practice wherein an individually tailored multidisciplinary program is formulated, which, through accurate diagnosis, therapy, emotional support and education, stabilizes or reverses both the physio- and psychopathology of pulmonary disease and attempts to return the individual to the highest possible functional capacity allowed by his pulmonary handicap and overall life situation.

The American Thoracic Society Statement on Pulmonary Rehabilitation published in 1981 highlights[5]: "In the broadest sense, pulmonary rehabilitation means providing good, comprehensive respiratory care for patients with pulmonary disease."

The newest definition of the PR process was developed by the National Institutes of Health Consensus Conference on Pulmonary Rehabilitation in 1994[6]:

> A multi-dimensional continuum of services directed to persons with pulmonary disease and their families, usually by an interdisciplinary team

TABLE 7–1
**CONDITIONS APPROPRIATE FOR
PULMONARY REHABILITATION**

Obstructive Pulmonary Disease

Chronic obstructive pulmonary disease (COPD)
Asthma
Asthmatic bronchitis
Chronic bronchitis
Emphysema
Bronchiectasis
Cystic fibrosis

Restrictive Pulmonary Disease

Interstitial fibrosis
Rheumatoid pulmonary disease
Collagen vascular lung disorders
Pneumoconiosis
Sarcoidosis
Kyphoscoliosis
Rheumatoid spondylitis
Severe obesity
Poliomyelitis

Other Conditions

Pulmonary vascular disease
Lung resection
Lung transplantation
Occupational/environmental lung diseases

Source: Reprinted with permission from Beytas, L and Connors, GL: Organization and management of a pulmonary rehabilitation program. In Hodgkin, JE, Connors, GL and Bell, CW (eds): Pulmonary Rehabilitation: Guidelines to Success, ed 2. JB Lippincott, Philadelphia, 1993.

of specialists, with a goal of achieving and maintaining the individual's maximum level of independence and functioning in the community.

Patient Selection and Sequence

In 1995, the American Thoracic Society published a document entitled *The Standards for the Diagnosis and Care of Patients with Chronic Obstructive Pulmonary Disease* (COPD) and, in an algorithm for the outpatient management of the COPD patient, includes PR in the therapeutic schema.[7] Patients with COPD are not the only patient population who benefits from PR. Restrictive pulmonary disease, pulmonary vascular diseases, lung resection, lung transplantation, occupational/environmental lung diseases, and long-term ventilation are also conditions appropriate for PR as seen in Table 7–1.

TABLE 7–2
**CRITERIA TO BE EVALUATED IN SELECTING A
PATIENT FOR PULMONARY REHABILITATION***

Effect of disease on patient's quality of life
Reduction in physical activity
Changes in occupational performance
Dependence vs. independence in activities of daily living
Effect of disease on the patient's psychosocial status (i.e., anxiety,
    depression, etc.)
Use of medical resources (i.e., hospitalizations, emergency room visits,
    etc.)
Presence of other medical problems
Assessment of pulmonary function
Any history of smoking
Motivation
Commitment to required time and to active participation in program
Transportation needs
Financial resources
Background

*Any patient with impairment because of lung disease and with motivation
should be a candidate for pulmonary rehabilitation.
Source: Reprinted with permission from Beytas, L and Connors, GL: Organization and management of a pulmonary rehabilitation program. In Hodgkin, JE, Connors, GL and Bell, CW (eds): Pulmonary Rehabilitation: Guidelines to Success, ed 2. JB Lippincott, Philadelphia, 1993.

PR is individualized to meet the needs of each patient. The sequence
of PR begins with patient selection and assessment of the patient's needs.
Any patient with impairment due to lung disease and with motivation
should be a candidate for PR. Other criteria to assist in selecting a patient
for PR are seen in Table 7–2.

Pulmonary function testing is very helpful in assessing a patient's lung
health, determining the extent of lung disease, diagnosing the lung disease,
and evaluating a patient for PR, although specific criteria for pulmonary
function abnormality should not be used alone in establishing patient eligibility for PR. The most important element is the effect of the disease on the
patient's quality of life. Is the disease causing any limitation for the patient,
other than just being present?

PR programs emphasize patient involvement and responsibility for the
patients' own health care. In selecting patients, it is important to assess
and document their willingness to actively participate in the rehabilitation
process. During all components of PR, the goals are to determine the "outcome" for the therapy provided. Documentation is necessary to reflect the
provided treatment program and for insurance reimbursement.

A patient's current smoking status is important to know but should not
be used as a denial for a patient's entrance into a PR program. In fact,
smoking cessation and nicotine addiction treatment should be a part of every

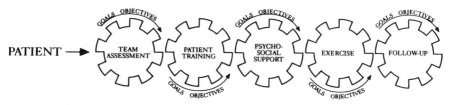

PATIENT →

GOALS OBJECTIVES
TEAM ASSESSMENT

GOALS OBJECTIVES
PATIENT TRAINING

GOALS OBJECTIVES
PSYCHO-SOCIAL SUPPORT

GOALS OBJECTIVES
EXERCISE

GOALS OBJECTIVES
FOLLOW-UP

FIGURE 7–1
The essential components of pulmonary rehabilitation are very specific. Once the initial assessment is completed, the foundation of the patient's individualized program is developed from the established goals and objectives. It is essential for each component to be incorporated into a comprehensive pulmonary rehabilitation program. *(From Connors, GL, Hilling, LR and Morris, KV: Assessment of the pulmonary rehabilitation candidate. In Hodgkin, JE, Connors, GL and Bell, CW [eds]: Pulmonary Rehabilitation: Guidelines to Success, ed 2. JB Lippincott, Philadelphia, 1993, with permission.)*

PR program. Other concurrent diseases or conditions may interfere with the rehabilitation process and need to be addressed, corrected, or stabilized prior to rehabilitation. Examples of the conditions that may be considered contraindications to PR are severe psychiatric disorders such as dementia or organic brain syndrome and significant or unstable medical conditions such as congestive heart failure, acute cor pulmonale, recent myocardial infarction, substance abuse, significant liver dysfunction, metastatic cancer, and disabling stroke.

Essential Components of Pulmonary Rehabilitation

To individualize a PR program to meet the needs of each patient, the essential components of PR must be followed. These components include assessment of the patient by each member of the PR team, patient training, psychosocial intervention, supervised exercise, and follow-up.[1] PR is *not* just an exercise or education program but a carefully integrated, comprehensive program that follows a logical sequence as seen in Figure 7–1. Table 7–3 takes these essential components and further expands them.

Assessment

The initial assessment lays the foundation for the PR program.[8] Evaluations by the program's director or coordinator, PR program physician, and exercise specialist will determine whether other team member assessments are needed. Other evaluations are made by allied health professionals such as an occupational therapist, nutritionist, and psychologist. The initial evaluation of the patient includes a history and physical examination as well as specific medical testing to determine or confirm the pulmonary diagnosis. Tests to be considered as part of the initial evaluation are listed in Table 7–4.

TABLE 7–3
**ESSENTIAL COMPONENTS OF A PULMONARY
REHABILITATION PROGRAM**

*Team Assessment**

PR medical director
Respiratory care practitioner
Nurse
Occupational therapist
Physical therapist
Exercise physiologist
Psychologist
Vocational counselor
Recreational therapist

Patient Training

Breathing retraining
Bronchial hygiene
Medications
Proper nutrition
Activities of daily living training
Panic control/relaxation
Energy conservation
Warning signs of infection
Sexuality for the pulmonary patient

Exercise

Exercise conditioning
Upper extremity strengthening
Respiratory muscle strengthening
Home program plan

Psychosocial Intervention

Support system and dependency issues
Anger management
Treatment of depression
Counseling
Coping styles
Self-efficacy for rehabilitation-related behaviors
Impact of role change

Follow-Up

Patient outcomes
Maintenance exercise group
Group meetings
Reevaluation as necessary

*An individualized pulmonary rehabilitation program will meet the specific
needs of the patient. Not every member of the pulmonary rehabilitation
program team may be involved with the patient. *Note:* Patient training or
exercise alone does not constitute a pulmonary rehabilitation program.
Source: Reprinted with permission from Beytas, L and Connors, GL: Organization and management of a pulmonary rehabilitation program. In Hodgkin, JE, Connors, GL and Bell, CW (eds): Pulmonary Rehabilitation: Guidelines to Success, ed 2. JB Lippincott, Philadelphia, 1993.

TABLE 7–4
**SUGGESTED TESTS DURING INITIAL EVALUATION OF
A PULMONARY REHABILITATION CANDIDATE***

Spirometry pre-/postbronchodilator
Lung volumes
Diffusing capacity
Chest radiograph
Resting electrocardiogram
Exercise test with cutaneous oximetry and/or arterial blood gas (simple or modified test such as
  6- or 12-min walk, calibrated cycle ergometer, or motorized treadmill)
Complete blood count
Basic blood chemistry panel

---

*It is acceptable to not repeat these tests if they have been done within 3 months before entering the pulmonary rehabilitation program or as determined by the pulmonary rehabilitation medical director.
Source: Reprinted with permission from Connors, GL and Hilling, L: Selection and team assessment of the pulmonary rehabilitation candidate. American Association of Cardiovascular and Pulmonary Rehabilitation: Guidelines for Pulmonary Rehabilitation Programs. Human Kinetics, Champaign, IL, 1993.

The comparison of previous test results with current tests is helpful in determining the impact and progression of the patient's disease. Often overlooked are problems with other systems, such as nasal/sinus, gastrointestinal, cardiovascular, neurological, or musculoskeletal. It is important to consider these body systems when outlining a comprehensive treatment program.[9]

A symptoms review should also be included in the assessment to identify conditions such as:

- Dyspnea
- Cough
- Sputum production
- Wheezing
- Hemoptysis
- Edema
- Chest pain

Other aspects to cover during the initial assessment are:

- Smoking status
- Environmental and occupational exposure
- Hobby or recreational exposure to pulmonary irritants
- Alcohol or drug history
- Prescribed medications and the patient's actual use of them
- Childhood pulmonary problems
- Family history of pulmonary disease

A physical examination is performed during the initial evaluation. This examination includes basic vital signs, use of accessory muscles on quiet

TABLE 7–5
OTHER TESTS TO CONSIDER FOR SELECTED PATIENTS

Maximal voluntary ventilation
Maximal inspiratory and expiratory pressures
Theophylline level
Pulmonary exercise stress test (metabolic study) with continuous ECG monitoring
Postexercise spirometry
Bronchial challenge (e.g., methacholine)
Cardiovascular test (e.g., Holter monitor, echocardiogram, radionuclide exercise stress test)
Polysomnography
Sinus radiographs
Upper gastrointestinal series
Skin tests

Source: Reprinted with permission from Connors, GL and Hilling, L: Selection and team assessment of the pulmonary rehabilitation candidate. American Association of Cardiovascular and Pulmonary Rehabilitation: Guidelines for Pulmonary Rehabilitation Programs. Human Kinetics, Champaign, IL, 1993.

breathing, neck veins, and extremity check for edema. The pulmonary physician may order additional tests on the patient based on the results of the initial assessment. Additional tests that may be ordered are listed in Table 7–5.

Assessment of nutritional status to determine the patient's need for weight reduction, weight gain, low-salt, low-cholesterol, or other specific dietary intervention is important. The assessment should include an evaluation of body weight, dietary history, and fluid intake.[10]

An exercise assessment, including an exercise test, should be carried out to determine whether hypoxemia occurs with activity or exercise, whether supplemental oxygen is indicated, whether orthopedic problems need to be addressed, and whether cardiac dysfunction is an issue. The type of exercise testing may vary, from a simple 6-min walk to a pulmonary exercise stress test with gas exchange measurements.[11] The exercise assessment is also useful in developing a home exercise program for the patient.

A psychological assessment should be included in the initial evaluation of the patient. The psychological assessment should evaluate for[12]:

- Depression
- Anxiety
- Anger management
- Effectiveness of the patient's rehabilitation-related behavior
- Coping style
- Family support and dependency issues
- Perception of stress
- General neuropsychological status
- Overall adaptation to disease
- Drug usage
- Compliance with the medical treatment prescribed
- The impact of role change due to disease

Various standardized questionnaires may be used for the assessment.[13] Psychotherapy and psychopharmacological agents as well as counseling and support therapy may be necessary for some patients.

Patient Training

Patient training involves the patient, significant other, and health care provider who is working with the patient. It is important that the patient know the status of lung health and the way in which medications, exercise, nutrition, relaxation, and other pertinent issues become essential to overall health status.[14] It is no longer acceptable for the patient to take a passive role in his or her health care. The patient must be involved to make behavioral changes that will lead to improved health. The specific issues to be addressed during a PR program will be individualized as determined during the initial assessment and may include the following[1]:

- Self-assessment
- Bronchial hygiene
- Activities of daily living
- Medications
- Respiratory modalities
- Exercise
- Psychosocial intervention

Table 7–6 details the specific components of the PR training sessions. The elements of the training sessions to be used are determined by the individual needs of each patient.

One of the primary goals of PR is to give patients the tools and knowledge to assist them in achieving the best possible quality of life. This goal can be accomplished by improving patient compliance with the treatment program and optimizing the role of prevention, for which patient training is essential.

Psychosocial Intervention

Living with a chronic lung disease is not easy. When the physician tells a patient with chronic lung disease that he or she must stop smoking, lose weight, exercise, take breathing medication daily and that, in spite of these measures, chronic lung disease cannot be cured, the common reactions are anger, depression, and anxiety. Psychosocial assessment is critical to identifying such problems and the need for specific treatment intervention.

Improving a patient's self-esteem, assisting the patient with adaptive coping skills, and teaching the patient to control or manage symptoms are essential to improving the patient's quality of life. Each team member has a role in addressing the psychosocial issues as related to his or her area of

TABLE 7–6
**PATIENT TRAINING CONSIDERATIONS IN
PULMONARY REHABILITATION**

Self-Assessment

- Anatomy and physiology of the respiratory system
- Disease process
- Knowledge of the medical tests ordered by the doctor
- Importance of avoiding environmental irritants
- Occupational lung hazards and cautions
- Principles of exercise and physical fitness
- Nutritional needs of the pulmonary patient
- Management of pulmonary symptoms
- Knowledge of trigger signals for the asthmatic
- Warning signals of an infection
- Prevention and vaccines (pneumococcal, influenzal)
- Avoidance of active and passive smoking
- Other specific considerations based on individual patient needs (i.e., pedal edema, sugar level, etc.)

Bronchial Hygiene Training

- Diaphragmatic breathing with pursed lip breathing
- Cough techniques
- Postural drainage therapy including positioning and percussion
- Positive expiratory pressure and autogenic drainage techniques

Activities of Daily Living Training

- Energy conservation techniques
- Leisure time activities
- Panic control and relaxation
- Sexuality
- Travel recommendations for the lung patient
- Community resources
- Vocational retraining

Medication Training

- Proper use, side effects, and role of medication in the treatment and prevention of lung impairment
- Proper use of aerosolized medications
- Medication changes during an acute exacerbation
- Proper medication dosing of the asthmatic when peak flows change

Respiratory Care Modalities

- Oxygen use
- Care and cleaning of aerosol devices
- Suctioning in the home
- Ventilator management in the home
- Sleep disturbances and equipment for treatment
- Home care issues

Psychosocial Training

- Coping with lung disease
- Stress management techniques
- Support system and dependency issues
- Anger management
- Depression treatment

expertise. Examples of psychosocial interventions are:

- Individual counseling
- Group support
- Biofeedback
- Stress management
- Panic control
- Family therapy
- Anger management
- Patient advocacy
- Community resources
- Durable power of attorney for health care
- Vocational counseling
- Home care follow-up
- Traditional psychotherapy
- Use of psychotropic medications such as antidepressants or relaxants

Exercise

Shortness of breath often leads to less activity. The reduced level of activity leads to greater shortness of breath. This cycle of deconditioning continues until interruption occurs. That interruption is exercise. Patients with chronic lung disease can improve their appetite, sleep better, enhance their tolerance of dyspnea, and achieve a higher level of work if exercise is included in their daily regimen.

The exercise specialist who is part of the PR team will outline an exercise program for the patient. This program is based upon the initial evaluation of the patient by the specialist. The patient may be evaluated for exercise with a 6-min walk with pulse oximetry, blood pressure, heart rate, and Borg scale determination, upper extremity strength measurements, or a pulmonary exercise stress test.

Regardless of the method used to evaluate the patient for exercise, four basic components always exist when prescribing a home exercise program: the mode of exercise, the intensity of exercise, the duration of exercise, and the frequency of exercise. The patient's mode of exercise will depend upon the exercise equipment available to him or her. This may include walking, swimming, riding a stationary bicycle, circuit training, or even weight training. The patient should be encouraged to choose the mode of exercise with which they feel most comfortable. Walking is often the best choice.

The intensity of exercise may be determined by using the target heart rate (THR). THR is $[0.6 \times (\text{peak HR} - \text{resting HR})] + \text{resting HR}$. For patients with very severe impairment, however, a THR may not be reliable. In such an event, the patient is instructed to exercise to a level of "perceived exertion." The patient must increase the intensity of the exercise program to achieve improved conditioning.

TABLE 7–7
FOLLOW-UP OPTIONS FOR PULMONARY REHABILITATION PROGRAMS

Regular physician visits
Maintenance exercise group
Program graduate group outings and trips
Program graduate group meetings
Referral to community groups (e.g., American Lung Association's Better Breathers Club)
Telephone follow-up by program staff
Newsletters
Postprogram questionnaires
Reevaluation as indicated
Home health referral
Home visits
National Pulmonary Rehabilitation Week (observed during the first week of spring)

Source: Reprinted with permission from Beytas, L and Connors, GL: Organization and management of a pulmonary rehabilitation program. In Hodgkin, JE, Connors, GL and Bell, CW (eds): Pulmonary Rehabilitation: Guidelines to Success, ed 2. JB Lippincott, Philadelphia, 1993.

The duration of exercise should be 20 to 30 min, at least three to four times per week. Interval training (breaking up the exercise session into shorter time segments) may be needed for the patient who is limited by dyspnea until the individual can work up to the 20- to 30-min goal. Some patients must be given a progression plan for their exercise program.

The initial exercise evaluation will have determined the patient's need for supplemental oxygen with exercise. Oxygen saturation of 88 percent or less during exercise training requires supplemental oxygen, with the liter flow titrated to achieve an oxygen saturation of 90 percent or above.

Follow-Up

The final component of PR is follow-up. The type of follow-up given to a participant varies from program to program. Patient compliance is improved when follow-up is a component of a PR program. Follow-up can assist the patient in reaching higher levels of long-term benefits. Examples of follow-up activities are listed in Table 7–7.

A follow-up program that has been incorporated into a PR program is also needed to determine the efficacy of a PR program. A follow-up program can evaluate patient outcomes, such as changes in exercise tolerance, to identify the efficacy of the program's components.[15] Tools used in evaluating patient outcomes are described in the list in Table 7–8.

Benefits of Pulmonary Rehabilitation

The benefits of PR are well documented, *but* the earlier a patient with mild lung impairment participates in PR, the more favorably the course of lung disease can be altered.[16] Some benefits of PR are[17]:

TABLE 7–8
EVALUATING PATIENT OUTCOMES

Changes in Exercise Tolerance
- Pre- and post 6- or 12-min walk
- Pre- and postpulmonary exercise stress test
- Review of the patient's home exercise training logs
- Measurement of strength
- Flexibility and posture
- Performance in specific training modalities (e.g., ventilatory muscle, upper extremity)

Changes in Symptoms
- Comparison of dyspnea measurements
- Frequency of cough, sputum production, or wheezing
- Weight gain or loss
- Psychological test instruments

Other Changes
- Activities of daily living
- Postprogram follow-up questionnaires
- Pre- and postprogram knowledge test
- Compliance improvement with pulmonary rehabilitation medical regimen
- Frequency and duration of respiratory exacerbations
- Frequency and duration of hospitalizations
- Frequency of emergency room visits
- Return to productive employment

Source: Reprinted with permission from Beytas, L and Connors, GL: Organization and management of a pulmonary rehabilitation program. In Hodgkin, JE, Connors, GL and Bell CW (eds): Pulmonary Rehabilitation: Guidelines to Success, ed 2. JB Lippincott, Philadelphia, 1993.

- Reduction in respiratory symptoms
- Reversal of anxiety and depression
- Improvement in ego strength
- Increase in ability to perform activities of daily living
- Improvement in exercise capacity and strength
- Improvement in quality of life
- Ability to continue or return to gainful employment (for specific patients)
- Reduction in the number of hospitalization days for patients with COPD
- Improvement in survival

The Respiratory Care Practitioner's Role in Pulmonary Rehabilitation

The RCP who chooses pulmonary rehabilitation as his or her workplace will find it very different from acute care. Although some patients may participate in PR while they are hospitalized, most PR clients participate in an outpatient program. Some aspects of PR, such as breathing retraining, symptom recognition, and energy conservation are often taught to inpatients who are not enrolled in a PR program. The home care RCP will use many of these components when working with the home care patient as well.

PR programs are held in a variety of locations. Many RCPs work in PR programs located within acute care hospitals or outpatient clinics. Some programs are held at local YMCAs or other exercise facilities. Some RCPs work with PR programs that are incorporated with cardiac rehabilitation programs.

The RCP participates in PR programs in many ways. The RCP may serve not only as a team member but often also as the program coordinator. As a member of the team, the RCP will conduct his or her part of the initial assessment on program participants and will attend team conferences to assist in developing an action plan for each patient. The RCP will also participate in the training sessions, giving lectures as well as one-on-one patient education. The RCP may be assigned the task of monitoring oxygen saturation during a 6-min walk or performing the pulmonary stress tests on participants. Some RCPs lead exercise sessions for the program participants.

RCPs who work with a pulmonary rehabilitation program must have exceptional assessment skills. This is especially important because they are evaluating many different aspects of the pulmonary patient, such as symptoms, medication review, psychosocial components, and exercise capability. The RCP must be capable of organizing and presenting information to groups of people. These groups may be not only PR programs but also Better Breathers clubs, senior citizens' and asthma support groups, state and local respiratory care organizations, and physicians.

RCPs must also be capable of organizing their thoughts well in written form. Documentation of assessments, action plans, and discharge summaries is essential for program reimbursement by insurance companies. RCPs may also assist with writing program materials that are distributed to the participants.

SUMMARY

Another venue for the RCP is pulmonary rehabilitation. Using assessment, education and training, and follow-up, the RCP can assist patients in improving their quality of life. The focus of the RCP is on the whole patient, not just on the pulmonary problem.

The RCP working with a PR program will emphasize *prevention* in every component of the program. The earlier a patient can participate in a program, the sooner he or she will learn to reduce or prevent pulmonary symptoms. This is very different from the acute care RCP's emphasis of *treatment*.

The home care RCP uses many of the components of PR when working with home care patients. The home care RCP can also reinforce patient education in a PR program during home visits. The home care RCP may evaluate breathing patterns, for example, when the patient uses the stairs in the home, in addition to reviewing the proper way to breathe during this exercise. Together, they may review panic control, energy conservation techniques, and coping issues. The PR RCP can work closely with the home care RCP when developing a home care program for the PR participant.

REFERENCES

1. Connors, GL and Hilling, L: American Association of Cardiovascular and Pulmonary Rehabilitation: Guidelines for Pulmonary Rehabilitation Programs. Human Kinetics, Champaign, IL, 1993.
2. Connors, GL: A primary role in secondary prevention. Respiratory Therapy Feb/March 1994, pp 31–34.
3. Macklem, PT and Permutt, S: The Lung in Transition between Health and Disease. Marcel Dekker, New York, 1979.
4. Petty, TL: Pulmonary Rehabilitation: Basics of Respiratory Disease, Vol 4. American Thoracic Society, New York, p 1, 1975.
5. Hodgkin, JE et al: Pulmonary Rehabilitation: Official ATS statement. American Review of Respiratory Disease 124:663, 1981.
6. Fishman, AP: Pulmonary rehabilitation research: NIH workshop summary. Am J Respir Crit Care Med 149:825, 1994.
7. American Thoracic Society: Standards for the diagnosis and care of patients with chronic obstructive pulmonary disease. Am J Respir Crit Care Med (suppl) 152:77, 1995.
8. Connors, GL, Hodgkin, JE and Asmus, RM: A careful assessment is crucial to successful pulmonary rehabilitation. J Cardpulm Rehabil 8:435,1988.
9. Branscomb, BV: Aggravating Factors and Coexisting Disorders. In Hodgkin, JE and Petty, TL (eds): Chronic Obstructive Pulmonary Disease: Current Concepts. WB Saunders, Philadelphia, 1987, p 183.
10. Donahoe, M and Rogers, RM: Nutritional assessment and support in chronic obstructive pulmonary disease. Clin Chest Med 11:487, 1990.
11. Ries, AL: The importance of exercise in pulmonary rehabilitation. Clin Chest Med 118:622, 1990.
12. Weaver, T and Narsavage, G: Physiological and psychological variables related to functional status in chronic obstructive pulmonary disease. Nurs Res 2:286, 1992.
13. Guyatt, G, Feeny, D and Patrick, D: Measuring health related quality of life. Ann Intern Med 18:622, 1993.
14. Celli, BR: Pulmonary rehabilitation in patients with COPD. Am J Respir Crit Care Med 152:861, 1995.
15. Ries, AL et al: Effects of pulmonary rehabilitation on physiologic and psychosocial outcomes in patients with chronic obstructive pulmonary disease. Ann Intern Med 122:823, 1995.
16. Petty, TL: Pulmonary rehabilitation for early COPD: COPD as a systemic disease. Chest 105:1636, 1994.
17. Fishman, AP (ed): Pulmonary Rehabilitation: Lung Biology in Health and Disease. Marcel Dekker, New York, Vol 91:3–817, 1996.

chapter 8

Respiratory Care in Alternate Sites

Janice Tucker, RCP, RRT

Subacute Care Facilities

Skilled Nursing Facilities

Rehabilitation Facilities

Respiratory Care Coverage in a Subacute or Skilled Nursing Facility

Indications for Respiratory Care
Respiratory Care Services
Requisite Skills
Documentation

Summary

Our population is growing older because people are living longer.[1] Many patients need specialized medical care and many depend on technical medical equipment. Although these patients are technology- or care-dependent, they do not need the level of care of an acute care facility. In addition, there is a strong focus on reduction of medical costs and provision of higher levels of care for lower levels of reimbursement. The combination of these factors—the need for a level of care higher than would be received at home and the need to provide that care at a lower cost to the health plans—has encouraged the rapid growth of subacute, rehabilitation, and skilled nursing facilities.[2] In fact, it is estimated that the subacute industry will grow from $2 billion a year in 1992 to $10 billion a year by the year 2000.[3] These facilities offer many opportunities for the RCP seeking employment outside the acute care facility. This chapter reviews the characteristics of these alternative sites and describes the role of the RCP in these facilities.

TABLE 8–1
**INTERDISCIPLINARY MEMBERS OF
THE SUBACUTE CARE TEAM**

Patient (and, at times, family members)
Physician
Nurse
Respiratory care practitioner
Physical therapist
Speech therapist
Occupational therapist
Dietitian
Social worker

Subacute Care Facilities

Subacute care is goal-oriented, comprehensive inpatient care designed for an individual who has had an acute illness, injury, or exacerbation of a disease process.[4] In general, the condition of an individual receiving subacute care is such that the care does not depend heavily on high technology, monitoring, or complex diagnostic procedures.

Subacute care is administered in various types of inpatient facilities. Some hospitals have special units or patient rooms designated for patients who require less than acute care. Some nursing homes also have units that are designated as subacute wards. There are free-standing subacute facilities, as well.

Subacute facilities are reimbursed by third-party payers, such as Medicare, quite differently than are acute care hospitals. For example, Medicare pays hospitals a fixed amount for a specific diagnosis regardless of the cost or the length of time it takes the hospital to provide that care. Subacute facilities are paid a daily rate for the care they provide as long as the patient requires it. This difference in payment systems encourages the hospital to move patients, especially Medicare beneficiaries, from acute care and into subacute care as early in the course of treatment as possible. Many hospitals have seen the financial advantage of developing on-site subacute units to keep patients within the hospital system while being reimbursed at a maximum level.

Subacute care requires the coordinated services of an interdisciplinary team, whose members are listed in Table 8–1. These team members work closely together to assess patients and to manage their specific medical needs. As stated earlier, these medical conditions require a higher level of care but not so high as to require acute care.

Some facilities call themselves subacute care facilities or claim they have a subacute care unit. Not every facility, however, meets the criteria as defined by the Joint Commission on the Accreditation of Healthcare Organizations (JCAHO). According to the JCAHO, seven factors are integral to the provision of subacute care[5]:

1. **Time:** Subacute care is rendered immediately after, or instead of, acute hospitalization.
2. **Reason for treatment:** Treatment will encompass one or more specific complex or unstable medical conditions.
3. **Caregivers:** The patient requires services that must be provided by a trained and knowledgeable interdisciplinary team. This team must be able to assess and manage specific medical conditions and perform necessary procedures for the patient.
4. **Site:** Subacute care is provided as an inpatient program.
5. **Frequency:** The patient's condition requires frequent (daily to weekly) assessment and review of the clinical course and treatment plan.
6. **Intensity:** The level of care is generally more intensive than that provided in a traditional nursing facility and less intensive than that of acute inpatient care.
7. **Duration:** The treatment lasts for a limited time or until the patient's condition stabilizes. A predetermined course of treatment is established that is specific to the individual patient.

Responsibilities of the RCP in the subacute care facility or unit are similar to those in the acute care setting. The RCP may perform maintenance ventilator care, ventilator weaning, and other "high-tech" procedures as well as routine procedures such as nebulizer therapy and breathing retraining. The RCP may work in a separate part of the hospital or go to a nursing home to work with patients. A key difference is the type of equipment available when the subacute facility is part of a nursing home and when it is freestanding. Freestanding subacute care buildings generally do not have piped-in oxygen or suction, so the RCP will be using oxygen tanks or concentrators and electrically powered suction machines and compressor-nebulizers. Diagnostic equipment such as blood gas machines and heart monitors are not usually standard equipment for these facilities, either, although hospital-based facilities do have these devices as well as laboratory and radiology services on-site. Oximetry is usually available.

The RCP is a key member of the subacute interdisciplinary team, participating in patient care conferences, family conferences, and discharge planning. The RCP also takes an active role in the comprehensive management of the patient's respiratory care. The RCP evaluates each new patient, determines an appropriate plan of treatment, and then communicates directly with the physician to establish goals. The RCP initiates therapy and trains the staff as needed for the continuation of therapy.

Skilled Nursing Facilities

A skilled nursing facility (SNF) is an institution (or part of an institution) that has a transfer agreement in effect with one or more participating hospitals and that is capable of providing inpatient skilled nursing care for injured, sick, or disabled persons. A transfer agreement is a written agreement providing for the transfer of patients between the hospital and the facility and for the interchange of medical information.[6,7] An SNF is also capable of providing rehabilitative services such as physical, occupational, speech, and respiratory therapy. Ancillary services like behavioral therapy, recreation therapy, and social and dietary services should also be available in an SNF. Other characteristics of an SNF are:

- It has policies (developed and periodically reviewed by a professional group, including a physician and a registered nurse) to govern skilled nursing care and related medical services.
- It has a physician, a registered nurse, or a medical staff responsible for the execution of such policies.
- It has a requirement that the health care of every resident must be under the supervision of a physician.
- It provides a physician to furnish necessary medical care in an emergency.
- It maintains clinical records on all patients.
- It provides 24-hour nursing service sufficient to meet the nursing needs in accordance with the policies developed by the facility.
- It provides methods and procedures for dispensing and administrating medications.
- It has a utilization review plan.
- It is licensed in accordance with the state and is approved by the state as meeting the licensing standards.
- It is in compliance with local, state, and federal health and safety requirements.

As with subacute facilities, some hospitals have an SNF on-site, but more frequently the SNF is a freestanding facility commonly referred to as a nursing home. SNFs do not usually have piped-in gases or suction, and the equipment used is often the same as that used in the home, such as liquid oxygen, oxygen concentrators, and compressor-nebulizers. An SNF offers a lower level of care than an acute or a subacute facility, most often providing convalescent or custodial care. The majority of SNFs do not have laboratory and radiology services or on-site physician coverage.

Responsibilities of an RCP in an SNF include many of the same respiratory modalities used in a subacute facility. Respiratory care procedures such as oxygen therapy, aerosol administration, and breathing retraining are the types of procedures the RCP performs in an SNF. Procedures are more limited, but the emphasis placed on patient assessment is often greater than that placed in venues in which the physician is always present. Physicians rely on accurate clinical information from the RCP to help them make decisions concerning treatment. Documentation is also an important part of the RCP's job, as the provided respiratory services must be justified.

Rehabilitation Facilities

Hospitals have struggled for a long time with the problem of technology-dependent patients who cannot be discharged because they lack a place to go. The hospital may have long ceased to receive payment for this patient's care yet continues to be responsible for providing it. Acute rehabilitation facilities have become the answer to many hospitals' discharge problems.[8]

Acute rehabilitation facilities are capable of providing a higher level of care than can be provided by a subacute facility. Patients sent to acute rehabilitation facilities must show some potential for rehabilitation as well as a need for that level of care. Patients admitted to these facilities must be capable of withstanding 3 hours of rehabilitation per day. For example, the ventilator-dependent patient must show some potential for weaning. The ventilator-dependent patient also requires monitoring and diagnostic testing (like blood gases) that are not available at the subacute facility.

Acute rehabilitation facilities may be located within hospitals or as stand-alone facilities. Medicare does not reimburse these facilities in the same manner as it reimburses acute care hospitals. Instead of reimbursing per diagnosis-related group (DRG), Medicare pays at a higher daily rate. Respiratory care services performed on patients in an acute rehabilitation facility are reimbursed within that per diem rate.

Many hospitals see that this payment system is financially lucrative and have designated part of their facilities to perform acute rehabilitation. Patients are transferred to the hospital's acute rehabilitation unit as early as possible during their hospital stay.

RCPs who practice in an acute rehabilitation facility find that their jobs are nearly identical to those in the acute care hospital. The level of care is high, and the RCP performs many of the same procedures as those performed in the intensive care unit (ICU). Some rehabilitation facilities have the ability to perform surgery, and most can provide laboratory and other diagnostic services on-site. The RCP is part of a team of health care professionals working to bring the patient to the highest level of function. Team effort is paramount.[9]

Respiratory Care Coverage in a Subacute or Skilled Nursing Facility

Medicare guidelines define respiratory care as those services prescribed by a physician for the assessment, diagnostic evaluation, treatment, management, and monitoring of patients with deficiencies and abnormalities of their cardiopulmonary function.[10] Respiratory care in these facilities is covered by Medicare Part A under the following criteria:

- The delivery of care must be furnished by a respiratory therapist who is employed by an acute care hospital that has a transfer agreement with the skilled nursing facility.
- Respiratory care services must be reasonable and medically necessary, based on the patient's current medical condition.
- Respiratory care services must require the skills of a licensed RCP (in states in which licensure is applicable). Services cannot be ordered for the convenience of the nursing staff. For example, if a stable tracheotomy patient is admitted to the SNF, the nursing staff should provide routine tracheostomy care. The RCP can be involved with setting up an education and training program for the patient and staff but cannot perform routine tracheostomy care once the training is completed.
- Respiratory care services must be ordered by a physician.
- Respiratory care services must be reasonable in terms of modality, amount, frequency, and duration.
- Respiratory care services must be generally accepted by the medical community as being safe and effective treatments for the purposes for which they are used.
- Respiratory care services are consistent with the nature and severity of the patient's symptoms and diagnosis.

Many medical conditions may indicate the need for respiratory care; to be covered under Medicare Part A, however, each patient's need for services and actual condition must be specified. Coverage of respiratory care services is not recognized by Medicare when performed on a mass production basis with no distinction made as to the individual's need and diagnosis for these services (for example, "standing orders"). Such orders are not covered because they lack individual distinction. Additionally, if respiratory care services are considered "routine," they are not reimbursable under Medicare Part A; rather, they are considered to be routine nursing care not requiring the skills of a licensed RCP.

TABLE 8–2
**DIAGNOSES AND TREATMENT
CONDITIONS THAT MAY INDICATE THE
NEED FOR RESPIRATORY CARE
PRACTITIONER SERVICES IN A SKILLED
NURSING FACILITY**

Chronic obstructive pulmonary disease
Atelectasis
Acute bronchitis
Bronchiolitis
Postoperative complications
Cystic fibrosis
Presence of an artificial airway
Laryngeal edema
Pneumonia
Acute respiratory failure
Inhalation injury

Indications for Respiratory Care

Table 8–2 indicates the types of diagnoses or treatment conditions that may indicate the need for skilled respiratory care services in an SNF. Respiratory care services must be ordered by the physician before the initiation of therapy. The physician's order must include the specific type of needed treatment and must contain the frequency and duration of therapy and the type and dosage of any respiratory medications to be administered.

Respiratory Care Services

RCPs practicing in a subacute or SNF perform many of the procedures that are used in the acute care hospital. The major difference is that not all the procedures performed in a subacute unit or SNF are recognized by Medicare as appropriate for skilled respiratory therapy reimbursement; consequently, the RCP may perform therapy for which the facility will not receive payment. Another difference is that respiratory care administered in these facilities is focused on *education and training* rather than on procedures. Table 8–3 outlines the types of respiratory care procedures performed by RCPs that are covered for payment by Medicare.

As Table 8–3 shows, the list of procedures performed by the RCP in these facilities is extensive. Intensive and emergency care procedures are not generally performed. The type of respiratory care that RCPs perform in these facilities is comparable to that given to patients on medical-surgical wards in a hospital that focuses on rehabilitation. Subacute facilities and SNFs are not set up to provide the type of care seen in ICUs and can usually provide only the most basic emergency procedures. Patients are assessed for emergent problems and sent to the acute care hospital for treatment.

TABLE 8–3
RESPIRATORY CARE SERVICES THAT ARE REIMBURSABLE BY MEDICARE WHEN PERFORMED BY RESPIRATORY CARE PRACTITIONERS

- Diagnostic testing for evaluation by a physician, such as basic spirometry and other pulmonary function tests; oxygen saturation testing by pulse oximetry; peak flow measurement; and sputum induction.
- Therapeutic use of ventilators and other respiratory care equipment, including noninvasive ventilation and resuscitation devices.
- Establishment and maintenance of artificial airways.
- Therapeutic use and monitoring of medical gases, including thorough documentation of the need for and effectiveness of therapy.
- Bronchial hygiene therapy including coughing, intermittent positive pressure breathing (IPPB), postural drainage, and chest percussion and vibration; nasotracheal and endotracheal suctioning; pulmonary rehabilitation techniques, including exercise conditioning, breathing retraining, and patient education regarding disease process; and periodic assessment and monitoring of acute and chronically ill patients for effectiveness of respiratory care services.

Requisite Skills

RCPs who choose acute rehabilitation, subacute, or skilled nursing care as a career path must be well versed in all respiratory care procedures. They must also be able to work well as part of the patient's care team, as this type of care is very team-oriented. Effective verbal and written communication skills are needed when working as part of a team.[11]

Exceptional assessment skills are necessary for the subacute or rehabilitation RCP. The RCP must be able to evaluate the patient by using the most basic of tools, as these facilities do not have all the monitoring devices found in an ICU. The RCP will use tools such as the stethoscope, the blood pressure cuff, and the oximeter to evaluate and make decisions about the patient's condition and treatment.

RCPs must also be able to view the patient differently than they might in the ICU. Subacute and long-term care are very outcome-oriented, so the RCP must consider each patient and establish *measurable* goals for him or her. Failure to establish these goals may result in failure to be reimbursed for the respiratory care of that patient.

The RCP must be a self-starter and an independent worker. That RCP may be the only RCP in the facility and must be able to get the work done and make good decisions without input from another RCP.

The RCP must have patience and compassion as well. Many patients in these facilities are there for a long time, and the RCP must develop a relationship with the person, not with the ventilator or the aerosol treatment. As in any setting, the RCP must treat the patient with dignity and respect.

Documentation

Another essential skill the RCP must possess is the ability to thoroughly document findings and services. The primary way to justify the care provided to the patient in the subacute facility or SNF is through meticulous documentation. The RCP will be performing an initial evaluation that includes obtaining the patient's medical history and chief complaint, signs and symptoms, results of a physical assessment, and diagnostic test results. An essential part of this evaluation is the determination of the patient's rehabilitation potential and the establishment of short- and long-term goals based on that potential. The RCP will then develop a care plan for the patient with these goals in mind.

The RCP also performs daily therapies on the patient, and these treatments must also be documented. Documentation must include the specific treatment data and medication ordered, the patient's heart and respiratory rate before and after therapy, breath sounds before and after therapy, and pertinent observations about the patient's subjective and objective response to therapy.

A weekly summary note describing the patient's outcome and response to treatment must also be completed by the RCP.[12] This summary must include any pertinent diagnostic testing information, including trends in oxygen saturation and peak flows. The summary should also include the current respiratory status of the patient, including any progress made during the week and justification for the need to continue or discontinue therapy. The RCP must include any recommendations for change in treatment or equipment needs.

Patients who meet their goals of treatment will have their therapy discontinued. When this occurs, the RCP is responsible for writing a discharge summary. The discharge summary includes the length of the treatment period, the reason for discharge, any discharge recommendations for follow-up treatment, and pertinent information regarding outcomes and response to therapy.

It becomes apparent that a large part of the RCP's job in the subacute facility or SNF is to properly document his or her work. This may be very different for the RCP who has spent a career working in the ICU filling out ventilator flow sheets.

SUMMARY

While respiratory care procedures are essentially the same in acute, subacute, and long-term care, key differences can be found in approach:

- The equipment is different. There may be no piped-in oxygen, and the equipment will be portable, electrically powered, and located at the bedside.

- There may not be immediate access to laboratory tests and radiographs.
- The physician may not see the patient on a daily or even weekly basis.
- There may not be around-the-clock RCP coverage; coverage might be for only 8 hours.

Patients in these facilities are called *residents* because the facility is considered to be their home. It may be temporary or it may be for the rest of their lives. Regardless of the length of time a patient may be a resident, the RCP is an invited guest in the patient's home. Some residents may not have any visitors other than the staff members for days, weeks, or ever. It is important for the RCP to be respectful, kind, and patient.

As hospitals continue to downsize, increasing numbers of RCPs will be seeking employment in these alternative facilities.[13] Not every practitioner is suited to working in long-term care, however. The RCP must be up to the challenge of working without "bells and whistles," have heightened clinical assessment skills, and like working with a real person, not a machine or a diagnosis.

REFERENCES

1. Giordano, M: Disease management of the older adult asthmatic patient. AARC Times 12:34, 1996.
2. Dunne, P: Demographics and financial impact of home respiratory care. Respiratory Care 4:309.
3. Bunch, D: Respiratory care career opportunities shift to alternate care sites. AARC Times 5:30, 1995.
4. Office of the Assistant Secretary for Planning and Evaluation: Subacute Care: Policy Synthesis and Market Arena Analysis. US Department of Health and Human Services, Washington, DC, Nov 1995.
5. Joint Commission on Accreditation of Healthcare Organizations: 1996 Accreditation Protocol for Subacute Programs. Oakbrook Terrace, IL, 1996.
6. Health Care Financing Administration: Medicare Intermediary Manual. US Department of Health and Human Services, (HCFA Pub 13-3, Section 3101.10 [c]), Baltimore, 1983.
7. Health Care Financing Administration: Code of Federal Regulations, Section 42, CFR 483.75 (N). US Department of Health and Human Services, Baltimore.
8. Taraszewski, R: Subacute respiratory care. Advance for Managers of Respiratory Care, 3:30–33, 1996.
9. Bunch, D: Phenomenal growth of subacute care offers new opportunities for RCPs. AARC Times 5:30, 1996.
10. Wiedeman, GT: Some RCPs jeopardize their careers and our future. Respiratory Care 1:123, 1995.
11. Daus, C: RCPs forge new ground in subacute care. Respiratory Therapy 2:87–88, 1995.
12. Toran, MR: Subacute care accreditation: Learning the ropes. The Case Manager 4:55–57, 1996.
13. Fowler, FJ and Machisko, FL: The emergence of subacute care. Home Health Care Dealer 1:59–64, 1995.

1

Common Home Care Procedures: Training Instructions

This section has been included to provide you with practical information about common respiratory home care procedures.

Following are sample patient instructions for equipment the home care RCP as an employee of most home medical equipment/respiratory therapy (HME/RT) companies is likely to set up. If you are a student planning to go directly into home care or a clinician already in practice, you can use these patient instructions to increase your knowledge of the way in which this equipment is actually used by patients in the home. Reviewing these sample instructions will also help you to understand the types of information home care patients should receive to use the equipment safely and properly.

Whether you are planning to work or already work in the acute or subacute care setting, you can also use these patient instructions to familiarize yourself with the differences in the equipment procedures from those in a hospital. Reviewing these sample instructions will better prepare you for use of this equipment when it is brought into the hospital before a patient's discharge.

Compressor-Nebulizer

Wash your hands before assembling nebulizer or measuring medications.
Assemble nebulizer if necessary.

1. Measure out medications or open a unit dose vial. Place the medications in the nebulizer.

2. Attach the tubing to the bottom of the nebulizer. Attach the other end of the tubing to the compressor, if necessary.
3. Turn on the compressor and place the nebulizer mouthpiece in your mouth. Breathe normally back and forth through the mouthpiece. You may take an occasional slow, deep breath during the treatment.
4. Tap the sides of the nebulizer periodically to loosen large droplets of medication so that they will drop to the bottom of the nebulizer bowl.
5. Continue to breathe the mist until the nebulizer begins to sputter and no more mist appears.

The treatment is complete when no medication remains in the nebulizer bowl.

Cleaning and Disinfection

1. Once a day, disassemble and wash the nebulizer parts (except the tubing). To wash the parts, place them in a small bucket or bowl dedicated for this purpose and wash in hot water and dish detergent.
2. Rinse the parts thoroughly in tap water, taking care to remove all traces of detergent.
3. Place the nebulizer parts on a clean towel to dry.
4. When the nebulizer parts are dry, assemble the nebulizer and store in a clean paper bag.
5. Every Monday, Wednesday, and Friday, disinfect your nebulizer after washing it in soap and water. Place the nebulizer parts in a solution of *1 part white vinegar to 3 parts tap water,* and soak them for 30 min. Rinse the parts thoroughly in tap water and place them on a clean towel to dry. Discard the vinegar solution after each use. You may also use a commercial disinfectant solution like Control III, but it is important to mix and use the solution exactly as the manufacturer recommends.
6. Assemble the nebulizer and store in a clean paper bag.

Troubleshooting

1. If your treatment is taking longer than usual or if you think the machine is malfunctioning, check that the tubing is securely attached to the compressor outlet and that the outlet is not leaking. You can also disconnect the tubing and use your finger to test the flow coming from the outlet. If the flow seems reduced, contact your HME company for machine replacement. You may have to use your metered-dose inhaler (MDI) until the machine is replaced.
2. If the compressor is not leaking at the outlet and the flow seems all right, check to be sure the tubing has no holes.
3. If there are no holes in the tubing, check the nebulizer to be sure the baffle is in place (if the baffle is removable).

4. If the nebulizer has been assembled properly, check to be sure the little "pinhole" jets are not occluded.
5. Try another nebulizer if you think the nebulizer might be the problem. If your troubleshooting efforts are unsuccessful, contact your HME company.
6. If your machine will not turn on, check the power cord to be sure it is plugged in, and check the light switch, if the outlet is controlled by one.
7. If your machine has been sitting in the cold, the compressor may have "frozen up." This can be corrected by flipping the power switch on and off several times until the compressor starts to work.

Helpful Hints

- Be sure to sit in a comfortable chair that allows you to sit up straight when taking your treatments.
- Many people find that taking their treatments before breakfast, before lunch, before dinner, and before bed is an easy way to remember the treatment schedule.
- It is helpful to time your daily activities after you have had your treatment and your lungs are most open.
- Keep at least one extra nebulizer on hand so you will have one to use while the other is being cleaned. It is also good to have an extra nebulizer on hand in case one breaks.
- You may find it useful to keep the same medication in MDI form to use when you are away from home and need a bronchodilator treatment. Your physician must prescribe this for you.
- Consult your physician if you experience any side effects from the medication, such as a racing pulse, headache, shakiness, or increased irritability. Also, consult your physician if the medication fails to make your breathing any easier.

Oxygen Concentrator

1. Your physician has ordered oxygen at _____ liters per minute to be used _____ hours per day. You should also use your O_2 at _____ liters per minute during exercise or exertion and _____ liters per minute during sleep. The oxygen will be administered via oxygen concentrator and nasal cannula.
2. The oxygen concentrator is an electrically powered machine that separates oxygen from the air in the room. The oxygen flow is regulated by a flowmeter on the front of the concentrator. *It is important that you not adjust the oxygen flow unless your physician has told you to do so.*

3. The oxygen passes through a long tube that is attached to a nasal cannula. The concentrator may not function properly if more than 50 feet of tubing is used. Place the concentrator in a location that will allow you to move about your home with 50 feet of tubing or less.

4. The concentrator should have 12 to 18 inches of clearance on all sides to allow for free airflow around the concentrator's cabinet. Do not place the concentrator against drapes or bedclothes, in closets, or near heater vents.

5. A bubble humidifier is usually not necessary if your oxygen flow rate is 4 liters per minute or less. A humidifier may be helpful, however, if you experience nosebleeds or dryness of the nose or mouth when wearing the oxygen. If a humidifier is used, it must be filled with distilled or boiled water, *not tap water.* The water will need replacement daily, and the humidifier will need cleaning and disinfecting.

6. The concentrator should be plugged into a grounded electrical outlet, if possible. Outlets that are not grounded increase the risk of electrical shock. Extension cords should not be used. Avoid plugging the concentrator into an outlet that is controlled by a light switch. If such an outlet is used, tape the light switch in the "on" position to eliminate the possibility of someone's accidentally turning the concentrator off.

7. A compressed oxygen cylinder will be placed in your home as a backup to your oxygen concentrator. The backup oxygen should be used only during electrical power outages or concentrator malfunction.

8. The concentrator has a foam filter that you must clean weekly. Pull the filter out and rinse it through with clean water to remove all traces of dust. Wrap the filter in a clean towel, squeeze it dry, and put it back in its holder. Failure to clean the filter weekly can cause the concentrator to overheat and stop working.

9. Use care when walking about your home to avoid tripping over the oxygen tubing.

10. Do not go within 6 feet of an open flame, and do not smoke while wearing your oxygen. Alert visitors to the use of oxygen in your home by placing a "No Smoking—Oxygen in Use" sign on your front door.

11. Avoid the use of petroleum products, hair sprays, and other combustibles when using oxygen.

12. Your concentrator requires periodic maintenance by the HME company. If you think it is time for maintenance, contact the company if it has not contacted you first.

Cleaning and Disinfection

1. If you are using a humidifier, empty and replace the water daily with distilled or boiled tap water.

2. Wash the humidifier jar and lid in hot water and dish detergent every Monday, Wednesday, and Friday. Use a container that is dedicated for this purpose.
3. Rinse the humidifier parts in clean tap water and then disinfect in a solution of *1 part white vinegar to 3 parts tap water.* Soak in the vinegar-water solution for 30 min.
4. Rinse the humidifier parts in clean tap water and place on a towel to dry.
5. Store the humidifier in a clean paper bag.
6. Replace your cannula or mask weekly and your oxygen tubing monthly.

Troubleshooting

- If your concentrator will not turn on, check the power cord to be sure that it is plugged in. Check the light switch if the outlet for the concentrator is controlled by a light switch.
- Check the circuit breaker on the concentrator. If it has popped out, turn the concentrator power switch off and push the circuit breaker back in. Turn the concentrator back on. If the circuit breaker pops out and the concentrator stops, switch to your backup oxygen source and contact your HME company.
- If your concentrator stops during use, it may be due to a power outage. If not, the concentrator may have overheated. Check to be sure the concentrator's cabinet has at least 12 inches of free space around it. Check the foam filter to see if it is clogged with dust; clean if necessary. Check the circuit breaker. If it has popped out, push it back in. If you are unable to determine the reason the concentrator has stopped, switch to your backup oxygen source and contact your HME company.
- If you feel you are not getting enough oxygen flow, put the nasal prongs in a glass of water to see whether bubbles are created. If no bubbles appear, check the oxygen tubing for kinks or occlusion.
- If no kinks or occlusions are found, check the humidifier (if one is being used) to verify that the jar and lid are screwed together tightly. Check the threaded connector to be sure that it is securely screwed onto the oxygen outlet and that it has not been cross-threaded. If the humidifier is malfunctioning, remove or replace it.
- If no problems with the tubing or humidifier are identified, switch to your backup oxygen source and contact your HME company.
- If you experience unusual shortness of breath that is not attributable to an infection or other medical problem, switch to your backup oxygen source and contact your HME company. Request that the company check the oxygen concentration being put out by your machine. If the oxygen concentration is too low, the concentrator will be replaced.

Liquid Oxygen System

1. Your doctor has prescribed oxygen at _____ liters per minute to be used _____ hours per day. You should also use your O_2 at _____ liters per minute during exercise or exertion and _____ liters per minute during sleep. The oxygen will be delivered via a liquid oxygen (LOX) system and a nasal cannula. Your doctor may have also ordered a portable LOX tank for you. The portable LOX tank is a small tank that you can fill yourself as frequently as you need to.

2. The LOX system uses a thermos-type container that is periodically filled with liquid oxygen by your HME company. The liquid oxygen, which is extremely cold, travels through warming coils that cause the oxygen to convert to gas. The oxygen passes through a flow control valve that is set to deliver the oxygen prescribed by your doctor. *It is important that you not adjust the oxygen flow unless your physician has told you to do so.*

3. The oxygen passes through a long tube that is attached to a nasal cannula. The LOX tank may not function properly if more than 50 feet of tubing is used. The LOX tank should be placed in a location that will allow you to move about your home with 50 feet of tubing or less.

4. The liquid oxygen in your LOX stationary tank is continuously evaporating at a slow rate. Consequently, you may hear a small amount of "hissing" from the tank, particularly if the HME company has just filled it or if your home is very warm. The LOX tank should not be put in an enclosed space like a closet, because the continuous evaporation creates an oxygen-enriched atmosphere that can be a fire hazard. The LOX tank should also be located at least 6 to 8 feet from any heat source or open flame.

5. A bubble humidifier is usually not necessary if your oxygen flow rate is 4 liters per minute or less. A humidifier may be helpful, however, if you experience nosebleeds or dry nose or mouth when wearing the oxygen. If a humidifier is used, it must be filled with distilled or boiled water, not straight tap water. The water must be replaced daily and the humidifier cleaned and disinfected periodically.

6. A contents gauge at the top of your LOX tank will tell you how much oxygen remains in the tank. Your HME company will have to come to your home to refill your stationary LOX tank; the frequency of refills depends on the size of the tank and your liter flow. The company will inform you of your delivery days.

7. Your portable LOX tank can be filled as often as necessary. The portable tank must be kept upright after filling; if the tank falls over, it will vent the oxygen and make a very loud noise. Secure the portable tank to prevent tipping and venting while transporting it in your car.

8. When filling the portable tank, watch it carefully and stop the filling

process once the tank is full to prevent overfilling and icing. Avoid skin contact with the liquid oxygen stream that appears in the vapor plume when filling; contact with liquid can cause a burn similar to frostbite.

9. Use care when walking about your home to avoid tripping over the oxygen tubing.
10. Do not go within 6 feet of an open flame, and do not smoke while wearing your oxygen. Alert visitors that oxygen is being used in your home by placing a "No Smoking—Oxygen in Use" sign on your front door.
11. Avoid the use of petroleum products, hair sprays, or other combustibles when using oxygen.

Cleaning and Disinfection

- If you are using a humidifier, empty and replace the water daily with distilled or boiled tap water.
- Wash the humidifier jar and lid in hot water and dish detergent every Monday, Wednesday, and Friday. Use a container that is dedicated for this purpose.
- Rinse the humidifier parts in clean tap water and disinfect in a solution of *1 part white vinegar to 3 parts tap water.* Soak in the vinegar solution for 30 min and discard the solution after each use. You may also use a commercially prepared disinfectant solution like Control III; follow the manufacturer's recommendations for mixing and discarding the solution.
- Rinse the humidifier parts in clean tap water and place on a towel to dry.
- Store the humidifier in a clean paper bag.
- Replace your cannula weekly and your oxygen tubing monthly.

Troubleshooting

- If you feel you are getting a reduced oxygen flow or the flow is absent, check the flow control valve to be sure it is set at the proper flow rate.
- If the flow control valve is set properly, put your nasal cannula in a glass of water and watch for bubbles. If no bubbles appear, check the oxygen tubing for kinks or occlusion.
- If no kinks or occlusions are found, check the humidifier (if one is being used) to verify that the jar and lid are screwed together tightly. Check the threaded connector to be sure that it is screwed securely onto the oxygen outlet and that it has not been cross-threaded. If the humidifier is malfunctioning, remove or replace it.
- If you cannot identify any problems with the tubing or humidifier, contact your HME company and request immediate evaluation and/or replacement.
- If you cannot turn the flow control valve or if it turns with great difficulty,

try pressing down on the plastic shroud covering the top of the tank while turning the flow control valve. Even if this maneuver works, contact your HME company and request immediate repair or replacement.

- If you experience difficulty disconnecting the portable tank from the stationary tank after filling, the filling connections have most likely frozen together. Leave the portable tank connected to the stationary tank for 10 to 20 min to allow the fill connection to warm up and thaw the connection. You can reduce the chance of freezing by drying both connections with a cloth before making the connection. You can also reduce the chance of freezing by avoiding overfilling.
- The contents of the portable tank will evaporate in about 24 hours if not used. Do not fill the portable tank until just before you use it; it may evaporate completely if you fill it the day or even the night before you plan to use it.
- If you experience unusual shortness of breath that is not attributable to an infection or other medical problem, request that your HME company check the flow rate and operating pressure of your tanks for accuracy.
- If your stationary tank hisses more than usual or for a much longer time than usual after it is refilled, notify your HME company.

Gaseous Oxygen Cylinders

- Your physician has ordered oxygen at _____ liters per minute to be used _____ hours per day. You should also use your O_2 at _____ liters per minute during exercise or exertion and _____ liters per minute during sleep. The oxygen will be administered via a gaseous oxygen cylinder and nasal cannula. Your physician may have ordered a tall stationary tank and/or a small cylinder system for portability.
- The oxygen cylinder contains pressurized oxygen. The cylinder may be made of steel or aluminum. The oxygen flow is regulated by a flowmeter attached to the regulator on top of the tank. *It is important that you not adjust the oxygen flow unless your physician has told you to do so.*
- The oxygen passes through tubing that is attached to the nasal cannula. The flow rate may be reduced if more than 50 feet of tubing is used. Place the oxygen cylinder in a location that will allow you to move freely about your home with 50 feet of tubing or less.
- The oxygen cylinder should be secured in a tank stand or cylinder collar at all times. Small cylinders should be laid on the floor when not kept in a cylinder cart. The cylinders should be placed at least 6 feet from heat sources or open flames.
- A bubble humidifier is usually not necessary if your oxygen flow rate is 4 liters per minute or less. A humidifier may be helpful, however, if you experience nosebleeds or dry nose or mouth when using the oxygen. If a

humidifier is used, it must be filled with distilled or boiled water, *not straight tap water.* The water must be replaced daily and the humidifier will need to be cleaned and disinfected. A humidifier should not be used with a portable cylinder.

- Use only the cylinder wrench or cylinder key provided with the equipment to open the oxygen tanks or change regulators. Do not use wrenches or other tools kept around the house. The tools used with oxygen cylinders must be oil-free.
- Use care when walking about your home to avoid tripping over the oxygen tubing.
- Do not go within 6 feet of an open flame, and do not smoke while wearing oxygen. Alert visitors that oxygen is being used in your home by placing a "No Smoking—Oxygen in Use" sign on your front door.
- Avoid the use of petroleum products, hair sprays, and other combustibles when using oxygen.

Cleaning and Disinfection

- If you are using a humidifier, empty and replace the water daily with distilled or boiled tap water.
- Wash the humidifier jar and lid in hot water and dish detergent every Monday, Wednesday, and Friday. Use a container that is dedicated for this purpose.
- Rinse the humidifier parts in clean tap water and disinfect in a solution of *1 part white vinegar to 3 parts tap water.* Soak in the vinegar solution for 30 min; discard the solution after each use. You may wish to use a commercially prepared disinfectant solution; if so, prepare, use, and store as recommended by the manufacturer.
- Rinse the humidifier parts in clean tap water and place on a towel to dry.
- Store the humidifier in a clean paper bag.
- Replace your cannula or mask weekly and your oxygen tubing monthly.

Troubleshooting

- If you feel you are getting low or no flow, check the flowmeter attached to the regulator to verify that it is set properly. Check the contents gauge to be sure the tank is not empty. Check the stem on the tank to be sure the tank has been opened to the regulator.
- If no problem can be identified at the tank, check the oxygen tubing for kinks or occlusion.
- If no kinks or occlusions are found, check the humidifier (if one is being used) to verify that the jar and lid are screwed together tightly. Check the threaded connector to be sure that it is screwed securely onto the oxygen outlet and that it has not been cross-threaded. If the humidifier is malfunctioning, remove or replace it.
- When putting a regulator on a new cylinder, if you experience leaks at

the yoke of the regulator, check to be sure a grommet is on the large pin that joins the regulator and the neck of the tank. Be sure that you have the two small pins lined up to the two holes on the neck of the tank. If the tank leaks from the stem when you turn the stem, contact your HME company for a replacement tank.

Continuous Positive Airway Pressure/Bilevel Therapy

- Your physician has prescribed nasal continuous positive airway pressure (CPAP)/bilevel therapy for you at _____ cm H_2O pressure. It will be used to treat your obstructive sleep apnea. You are to use it whenever you sleep. The CPAP/bilevel device blows air through a mask you wear on your nose.
- Place your CPAP or bilevel machine at your bedside. You can set it on a bedside table, on the floor, or in any location that suits you. You can use up to 12 feet of tubing between the machine and your mask.
- Wash your face each night before putting on your nasal mask. If ordered, use your saline or prescription nasal spray prior to putting on your mask. *Do not use over-the-counter nasal decongestant sprays for more than 2 days without first checking with your physician. Do not insert petroleum jelly or mentholated petroleum jelly into your nose.*
- You may not tolerate wearing your CPAP or bilevel device all night right away. Wear it as long as you can, trying to increase your use time each night. The goal is to wear the device all night as soon as possible.
- It is not necessary to tighten your headgear straps as much as you can; rather, adjust the mask as loosely as possible without feeling any leaks, particularly near your eyes. Overtightening the straps can cause the mask to create pressure sores on your face.
- If you experience head congestion, an uncomfortably dry mouth, nasal irritation, or nosebleeds, you may benefit from a cool or heated passover humidifier. If using a humidifier, you must use distilled or boiled tap water to fill it; do not use straight tap water. You must also clean and disinfect the humidifier and long tubing every day.
- Once you are able to wear your CPAP/bilevel device all night, you should begin to feel better. Most CPAP wearers report that they wake up feeling refreshed and without morning headaches. They report that they do not feel tired during the day and do not need to take naps as they did before starting the therapy. If you do not feel better after 2 or 3 weeks of consistent CPAP use, contact your physician or sleep lab.

Cleaning and Disinfection

- Your mask should be washed daily with dish detergent or liquid hand soap as recommended by the manufacturer.

- Your headgear should be hand-washed and air-dried weekly or more frequently if necessary.
- Your tubing should be washed once a week in dish detergent and hot water. The tubing should be hung to dry. Hanging the tubing in your bathroom is not recommended, as it can become contaminated from the spray caused by flushing your toilet.
- If you are using a cool or heated humidifier, disassemble and wash the humidifier parts, including the long hose, in dish detergent and hot water *daily*. Rinse the parts and tubing in tap water and disinfect in a solution of *1 part white vinegar and 3 parts water,* soaking the parts for 30 min. If recommended by the manufacturer, the humidifier may be placed in the dishwasher. As an alternative, you may use a commercially prepared disinfectant solution like Control III; however, be sure to prepare, use, and discard it according to manufacturer's recommendations.
- If your machine has a foam filter, rinse it weekly in tap water, place it in a towel, and squeeze it dry. If your machine has an ultrafine paper filter, replace it once a month. For other machines, change or replace the filters according to the manufacturer's directions.

Helpful Hints

- If the air from the machine feels cold on your nose, put the long hose attached to your mask under your blankets. Your body heat will warm the hose and make the temperature of the air more comfortable. A heated humidifier can also help this problem.
- If you wake up and find air coming out of your mouth or if your mouth is excessively dry, you may need to use a chin strap. Report these problems to your HME company or sleep lab.
- You may experience some soreness at the bridge of your nose when first getting used to the mask. Placing a small piece of moleskin or "artificial skin" on this area will protect it from further irritation.
- If you experience a lot of "rain-out" in the long hose when using a humidifier, it is helpful to put the CPAP machine and humidifier on the floor or at least at a lower level than your bed.
- Some CPAP users report waking up with a sore back. This is because they lie still during the night. If you experience this, you should expect it to improve as you adjust to the therapy; if it is very uncomfortable, consult your physician.
- Sinus and ear pain are common during CPAP use; however, these problems must be treated. Consult your physician, who may prescribe a decongestant or antibiotic for you.
- CPAP and bilevel machines should be taken when traveling and even when camping. Contact your HME provider for information on making the power adaptations when traveling abroad or when camping.

Apnea Monitor

- Your physician has prescribed an apnea monitor for your baby. This device will monitor your baby's breathing and heart rate and will alarm if they are not within the limits the doctor has prescribed. *An apnea monitor will not prevent events from occurring but, if used properly, it will alert you to those events. It is important to be trained in infant CPR before going home with your baby.*
- You should use the apnea monitor whenever your baby is sleeping or when you are not holding him or her. Many babies fall asleep when riding in a car, so take the monitor with you.
- The apnea monitor will run on an internal battery. It is important to keep the monitor plugged in as much as possible to keep the battery charged. You should use the battery only when you are away from an electrical outlet or during power outages.
- Place the apnea monitor at least 6 feet away from electrical appliances. Do not place an intercom or portable telephone near the monitor, and do not place the monitor on top of an electric blanket.
- The rubber or stick-on electrodes should be placed under your baby's armpit at nipple level. Improper placement can lead to erroneous or equip- ment alarms. Do not use oil, creams, or powder on the areas in which the electrodes will be placed, as they can interfere with the electrode's monitoring ability.
- The rubber electrodes should be affixed to the electrode belt and wrapped snugly around the baby's chest; you should be able to fit only two fingers under the electrode belt if it is wrapped properly.
- It is helpful to run the two lead wires out of the foot of the baby's clothing to keep them away from the baby's head and neck.
- It is helpful to keep a record of alarms that occur. Record such information as the time of day, whether the alarm was human or equipment-related, any physical changes in the baby, and the action you took to correct the alarm. Take this record with you to the baby's medical appointments. Your physician may find this record helpful in identifying any trends in events.
- Always keep a spare set of electrodes and lead wires with you in case of problems; you do not want the monitoring interrupted while you are awaiting delivery of supplies.

Cleaning and Disinfection

- The rubber electrodes should be cleaned daily with soap and water. This is easily remembered and accomplished if you clean them when you bathe your baby. Do not scrub the electrode surface with a washcloth, as this can abrade the electrode and interfere with conduction.

- If using stick-on electrodes, replace them when they begin to lose their stickiness. Clean the baby's skin to remove any adhesive that may remain before applying new electrodes.
- The electrode belt should be hand-washed and air-dried weekly or more frequently if needed.

Responding to Alarms

- Your monitor will make a "beeping" sound if responding to breathing or heart rate that is outside the set limits. The monitor will make a continuous sound if it is responding to a problem with its monitoring ability.
- If you hear a beeping sound, wait a few seconds to see if the problem corrects itself. The alarm sound may stimulate the baby, correcting the alarm situation. If the problem does self-correct, look at the monitor to see which alarm light remains lit. The doctor may want you to record these alarms.
- If the problem does not self-correct, the beeping will continue. Check your baby's color and observe him or her for breathing. You can try to stimulate the baby by stroking the cheek or the bottoms of the feet. You may need to pick up the baby for additional stimulation.
- If the baby does not appear to be breathing, call 911 and then initiate CPR.

Troubleshooting

- If you get a "loose connection" alarm, start with the baby and work your way back to the monitor. Check the electrode belt to verify that it has not slid up or down on the baby's chest. Check the belt's snugness. Be sure the electrodes are still on the baby's sides under the armpit at nipple level.
- If adjusting the electrodes or electrode belt does not correct the problem, look at the electrodes to see if they have a buildup of dead skin or other debris on them. Clean the electrodes. If they do not appear soiled, rub some tap water into them with your fingers to increase their conductivity. Replace the electrodes, if necessary.
- If the electrodes do not seem to be the problem, check the lead wires to verify that they are properly plugged into the patient cable. Change the lead wires, if necessary.
- Check the connection between the patient cable and the monitor.
- Verify that the monitor is plugged into an electrical outlet.
- If you cannot locate the problem after following these steps, contact your HME company.
- If you get "human" alarms that you feel are erroneous, follow the previous steps.

Suction Machine

1. Your physician has ordered a suction machine to help you with airway clearance. You will be using the suction machine to aspirate secretions from your mouth and throat or your trachea. You will be using a _____ tonsil (Yankauer) tip or _____ suction catheter.
2. The suction machine uses an electrically powered vacuum device with a collection bottle. The suction pressure is adjustable; you should adjust the pressure to no more than _____ mm Hg. Setting the pressure too low will result in ineffective clearance of secretions. Setting the pressure too high can result in trauma to the tissues in the oropharynx or trachea.
3. Before beginning the suction procedure, it is important to *wash your hands.* You may wish to wear gloves if suctioning the trachea.
4. Keep a small container nearby that you can fill with distilled or boiled tap water. It will be used to suction through the tonsil tip or catheter to clear it of secretions. Do not leave water sitting in the container if you are using suction catheters, but instead fill it just before suctioning.
5. Turn on the suction machine and advance the tonsil tip or suction catheter to the back of the throat. Avoid causing yourself (or the person you are suctioning) to gag, as it can cause vomiting and possible aspiration. Sweep the tonsil tip or catheter from one side of the mouth to the other. If the person being suctioned will not open the mouth, insert the tip or catheter into the corner of the mouth and move it along the teeth to the back of the mouth.
6. If suctioning the trachea through a tracheostomy tube or laryngectomy stoma, limit the suctioning period to 10 to 15 sec. Do not cover the thumb port on the catheter until you have advanced the catheter into the trachea. Advance the catheter until you feel resistance and then back it off a small distance before applying suction. Rotate the catheter with your fingers while quickly withdrawing it.
7. Suction water through the tonsil tip or catheter after each suctioning pass.
8. At the conclusion of the suctioning procedure, suction water through the tonsil tip or suction catheter. Suction air through the tonsil tip, and suction air through the catheter if it is going to be used again. Place the tonsil tip or suction catheter into a paper bag until it is needed again.
9. *Wash your hands after suctioning, even if you wore gloves.*

Cleaning and Disinfection

1. The collection bottle should be emptied at least once per day and every 8 hours or more if the person is being suctioned frequently. The contents should be emptied into the toilet. Failure to empty the suction bottle

before it becomes full can result in interruption of the suction pressure and possibly damage to the suction machine.

2. Periodically suction a solution of 50 percent hydrogen peroxide and 50 percent water through the suction catheter, tonsil tip, and suction connecting tubing to help remove debris.

3. Wash the suction collection bottle with dish detergent and hot water every other day. You may wish to wear gloves when handling the collection bottle. Use a bottle brush to scrub debris away from the sides of the bottle.

4. Replace the tonsil tip and suction connecting tubing once a week or more frequently if necessary.

5. Replace the suction catheter once per day or more frequently if necessary.

Troubleshooting

- If you feel you are not getting enough suction pressure, try suctioning water through the tonsil tip or catheter. Check the suction pressure setting of the vacuum gauge and adjust, if an adjustment is needed.
- Check the collection bottle to verify that the lid is on properly and that no ports are open on the lid.
- Check all tubing connections. Replace tubing if necessary.
- Replace the hygroscopic filter if the suction machine has one.
- If these steps do not correct the problem, contact your HME company.

2

Case Reviews

The following case reviews illustrate the types of patients and situations that are often encountered during home visits. These reviews are taken from actual situations and patients encountered by the authors. They serve to illustrate the diversity of experiences the home care RCP can have from day to day and from patient to patient.

The common thread throughout these case studies is *problem solving*. The home care RCP performs the necessary assessments and uses the information to identify the patient's problems or needs. An action plan is then established to correct the problems or meet the needs. It is important to recognize that problems are identifiable not only during the initial visit but can also be found during subsequent visits and even during telephone follow-up.

Students can use these case studies to help open their eyes to see patients in many different ways. The home care RCP is not limited to listening to lungs and taking pulses. Although it is extremely important, the physical assessment is not the only type of assessment to be made on the home care patient. The student can use these case studies to learn to look for clues in other areas, such as the physical environment, other caregivers, or even financial issues. After reading the case presentation, the student should try to identify as many problems as he or she can and propose an action plan to solve each problem.

Case Review #1

Mrs. Webster is a 68-year-old woman who has been under a physician's care for chronic obstructive pulmonary disease (COPD). During her last clinic visit her physician ordered home oxygen for her. Her prescription was for 2 liters per minute (L/min) via nasal cannula, and the oxygen was to be worn during exercise or exertion. A liquid oxygen (LOX) system was set up for her.

An initial visit was made by the home care RCP. Mrs. Webster lives in a single-level, very clean home with her husband. Her small grandchildren live next door and visit frequently. Mrs. Webster is a very active woman who is co-owner of a catering business, and she is adamant about being able to work as much as she can. She feels the oxygen will limit the amount of time she can be away from home while catering. She admits that wearing oxygen is cosmetically unappealing to her and a real nuisance but also admits she feels better when she wears it. She tends to put it on *after* she completes an activity that makes her short of breath.

An evaluation of her physical environment shows her home to be safe and appropriate for home oxygen equipment. A "No Smoking" sign is posted at the entrance of the house. Mrs. Webster must climb three steps to go from the garage into the house. The stationary LOX tank is placed in a spare bedroom that is centrally located.

Physical assessment shows Mrs. Webster's blood pressure to be 125/80 mm Hg, her heart rate is 91 and regular, and her respirations are 18 per min. Her breath sounds are decreased. She has slight swelling in her ankles. Her room air oxygen saturation at rest was 94 percent, and, after she had ambulated for 5 min, it dropped to 88 percent. Mrs. Webster says she does not cough, and she uses an albuterol inhaler when she remembers it, although the prescription is for four times per day.

Problem #1

This patient is not compliant with her oxygen prescription.

GOAL

Mrs. Webster will wear her oxygen with exercise and exertion as prescribed.

Mrs. Webster agrees to try an oxygen conserving device (OCD) system. A follow-up visit is scheduled to instruct her in the use of this system and to evaluate her oxygen saturation during some of her activities while on the system.

Activity/Service

- Review with patient the indications for supplemental oxygen and the signs, symptoms, and physical effects of hypoxemia.
- Review the meaning of "with exertion and exercise" (eating, dressing, performing housework, walking, shopping, working at her catering business).
- Suggest using an OCD, in particular, one that is built into a small, portable LOX tank. This would allow Mrs. Webster to be away from home for

significantly longer periods. It would also allow her to use the oxygen more consistently, rather than keeping the tank in the car and going out for "hits" of oxygen when she has a chance.

Problem #2

The patient is not compliant with her inhaler use.

GOAL

Mrs. Webster will use her albuterol inhaler four times per day as prescribed.

Activity/Service

- Review indications and benefits of consistent inhaler use.
- Observe the patient's technique and reinstruct as necessary.
- Encourage her to use a "before breakfast, before lunch, before dinner, and before bed" schedule as an easy way to remember to use the inhaler.

Mrs. Webster agrees to use the schedule for her metered-dose inhaler (MDI). We will review her progress during the next home visit.

Case Review #2

Mrs. Washington is a 74-year-old woman diagnosed 6 months ago with amyotrophic lateral sclerosis (ALS). She is in the hospital pending discharge and will need home oxygen and a suction machine for oral suction. She will also require a hospital bed and seat lift chair. Her husband is to be her primary caregiver, and her three daughters will take turns providing respite care.

As of this time, the ALS has affected only Mrs. Washington's extremities and her ability to swallow. She is able to ambulate with the use of a wheeled walker but cannot pick up her feet more than 1 or 2 inches She tires fairly quickly because of the muscle weakness. She has a gastrostomy tube in place and is fed enterally by 60-cc syringe bolus feed. She is discouraged from taking anything but ice chips by mouth.

As part of the discharge planning team, the home care RCP evaluates Mrs. Washington's home to determine its appropriateness for her equipment needs. Her home is a very old three-story Victorian with old wiring. She is going to be living in the present dining area so that she can be with her family as much as possible. The home is wired with only three circuits, and one circuit supplies electricity for the kitchen, dining area, and living room. The circuit supports all the kitchen appliances, a television and VCR, and several lamps.

The floors are covered with wall-to-wall carpeting. On top of the carpet are oriental rugs, and on top of the rugs are plastic floor runners. Neither the rugs nor the plastic floor runners are secured to the floor in any way. Both exits from the home require descending very steep staircases.

Problem #1

The home's electricity may not be adequate to handle the additional load of the hospital bed, seat lift chair, oxygen concentrator, and suction machine. Mrs. Washington's progressive disease will likely require her to use additional equipment in the future, perhaps even a home ventilator.

GOAL

The patient and her family will be able to operate the necessary equipment safely while continuing to operate the household appliances.

Activity/Service

- Recommend that an electrician evaluate the home's wiring.
- Recommend that the home be wired with a dedicated circuit for the medical equipment in the proposed living area.

Problem #2

The uneven surfaces created by the plastic runners on top of the rugs that sit on the carpeting will pose a hazard for the patient when she tries to ambulate with her wheeled walker.

GOAL

Patient will be able to move freely and safely about her living area with her walker. The floor coverings will not impede her or create a hazard.

Activity/Service

- Recommend that the plastic runners and rugs be removed from her living area.
- Recommend that a physical therapist evaluate the home.

Problem #3

The home's exits will be extremely difficult for the patient to use, particularly in an emergency.

GOAL

The patient will be able to quickly and safety exit the home in an emergency.

Activity/Service

- Devise an emergency exit plan. The patient will have to be placed on a chair and carried down the staircase whenever she leaves the home. She may need to be strapped into the chair to keep her secure as her muscles become progressively weaker. The physical therapist will be asked to provide training for all caregivers in transporting the patient by chair and in proper body mechanics.

Case Review #3

A routine home visit was made for an oxygen patient, a 61-year-old man with asbestosis and COPD. Mr. James has been notorious for trying to wean himself off the oxygen against the orders of his physician. Mr. James lives with his wife, son, and daughter-in-law; all three essentially ignore him. He provides his own care the best that he can.

Today Mr. James complains of having been short of breath for 2 or 3 days "or maybe it's been more like a week." His oxygen is turned up to 4 L/min, although his prescription is for 2 L/min. He has not informed his doctor of his increased shortness of breath.

Physical assessment reveals that his blood pressure is 160/100 mm Hg, and his heart rate is 123. His respiratory rate is 32, and his oxygen saturation is 78 percent on 4 L/min. He is diaphoretic and very warm to the touch. He denies cough or sputum production but is bringing up copious amounts of green secretions during the home visit. Mr. James appears to have been incontinent of urine and states that he has been too short of breath to walk to the bathroom.

Problem

This patient is seriously ill and is not being cared for by his family.

Activity/Service

Call 911 for ambulance transport to the nearest emergency room.

Case Review #4

A home visit is made to set up a compressor-nebulizer for an 80-year-old woman with chronic bronchitis. Mrs. Smith lives alone in an apartment complex for senior citizens. Her next-door neighbor looks after her and is there with her to learn about using the equipment.

Mrs. Smith will be taking her treatments at the kitchen table, so the compressor is placed there. Her electrical outlet is grounded. She can assemble the nebulizer but has difficulty attaching the tubing to the nebulizer and compressor.

She brings out the medication the doctor has prescribed for her treatments, which she is supposed to take every 4 to 6 hours. The medication is unit dose albuterol and comes in little bottles with tiny, twist-off caps. Mrs. Smith has arthritis in her hands and cannot open the unit dose bottles. Mrs. Smith will be able to clean and disinfect the nebulizer as instructed but, again, she has difficulty disconnecting the tubing from the nebulizer.

Problem #1

Mrs. Smith is unable to open her unit dose medication bottles.

GOAL

She will be able to take the treatments as prescribed.

Activity/Service

- Arrange with Mrs. Smith's neighbor to have her come over each morning to crack open each unit dose vial that will be needed that day. Once the seal is cracked, Mrs. Smith will have no trouble getting the top off the vial.
- Leave instructions for Mrs. Smith to request unit dose albuterol in plastic vials with pull-off tops from her pharmacy when it is time for her to get her prescription refilled.

Problem #2

Mrs. Smith is unable to connect and disconnect the nebulizer tubing.

GOAL

Mrs. Smith will be able to assemble and disassemble the nebulizer without assistance.

Activity/Service

- Provide patient with a permanent nebulizer with a thumb port connection. This thumb port connection will be easy for her to connect and disconnect from the nebulizer. Review use of thumb port and remind patient that this nebulizer will not work unless the thumb port is covered.
- Review assembly, disassembly, and cleaning of the permanent nebulizer.

Follow-Up Plan

- A telephone follow-up is scheduled. Mrs. Smith is encouraged to call with any questions or problems she may have in taking the treatments. A home visit will be made if the telephone follow-up identifies any problems.

Case Review #5

Mr. Boggs is a 43-year-old man recently diagnosed with obstructive sleep apnea. His physician has ordered continuous positive airway pressure (CPAP) at 12 cm H_2O pressure during hours of sleep. Mr. Boggs does not agree with the diagnosis and denies having any symptoms. He states he is willing to try CPAP therapy only to placate his wife.

A home visit is made to set up and teach the patient to use the CPAP machine. Mr. Boggs complains of feeling claustrophobic during the CPAP titration phase of the sleep study. He also states he has chronic sinus problems for which he uses over-the-counter decongestant nasal sprays, something he has done regularly for several years. He complains that he will no longer be able to travel or go camping in his recreational vehicle if he uses the CPAP.

Problem #1

Mr. Boggs has not "bought in" to his diagnosis.

GOAL

He will use the CPAP during hours of sleep as prescribed.

Activity/Service

- Review physician's prescription and indications for CPAP.
- Review the positive changes Mr. Boggs will experience with consistent CPAP use.
- Provide him and his wife with educational support materials to read.
- Encourage patient to participate in the local CPAP support group.

Problem #2

Mr. Boggs complains of claustrophobia, which can make it difficult to tolerate a CPAP mask.

GOAL

Patient will tolerate wearing the CPAP mask all night, every night.

Activity/Service

- Show patient several different types of facial appliances and allow him to try each one while hooked up to the CPAP machine.
- Remind patient of the control he has and encourage him to take off the mask as needed until he becomes used to it.
- Obtain physician approval to initiate the "ramp" feature on the CPAP machine and demonstrate to the patient that he will be able to fall asleep with the CPAP pressure at a low setting. The machine will gradually increase the pressure to the preset therapeutic level over a period of minutes and he will not be aware that it is happening. Encourage the patient to voice his concerns and complaints.

Problem #3

Patient has chronic sinus problems.

GOAL

He will tolerate the CPAP with minimal sinus irritation.

Activity/Service

- Encourage the patient to switch to a saline nasal spray and to use it just before bed and as needed during the daytime to lubricate his nasal passages.
- Strongly encourage the patient to discuss his chronic use of nasal decongestant sprays with his physician.
- Provide patient with a cool or heated in-line humidifier for use with the CPAP.

Problem #4

Patient wants to travel, go camping.

GOAL

He will be able to travel whenever he wants without interrupting his CPAP therapy.

Activity/Service

- Provide Mr. Boggs with information on the operation of his CPAP equipment with 110-volt, 220-volt, or 12-volt power.
- Instruct him in hooking up his CPAP to a cigarette lighter or 12-volt battery.

- Review airline travel with the CPAP machine.
- Encourage the patient to travel as often as he wishes.

Follow-Up Plan

- Telephone follow-up after the first night of treatment. Home visits for mask refit as needed. Weekly telephone follow-up until patient is using CPAP all night. Follow-up prn from that point.

Index

A number followed by an "f" indicates a figure; a number followed by a "t" indicates a table.